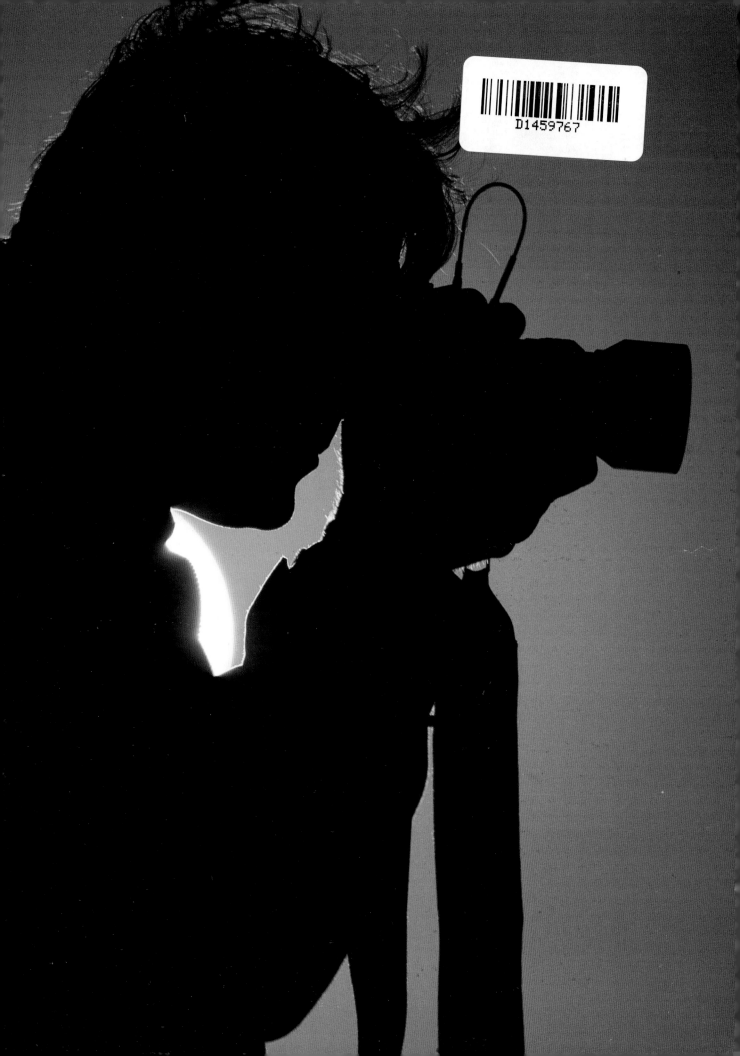

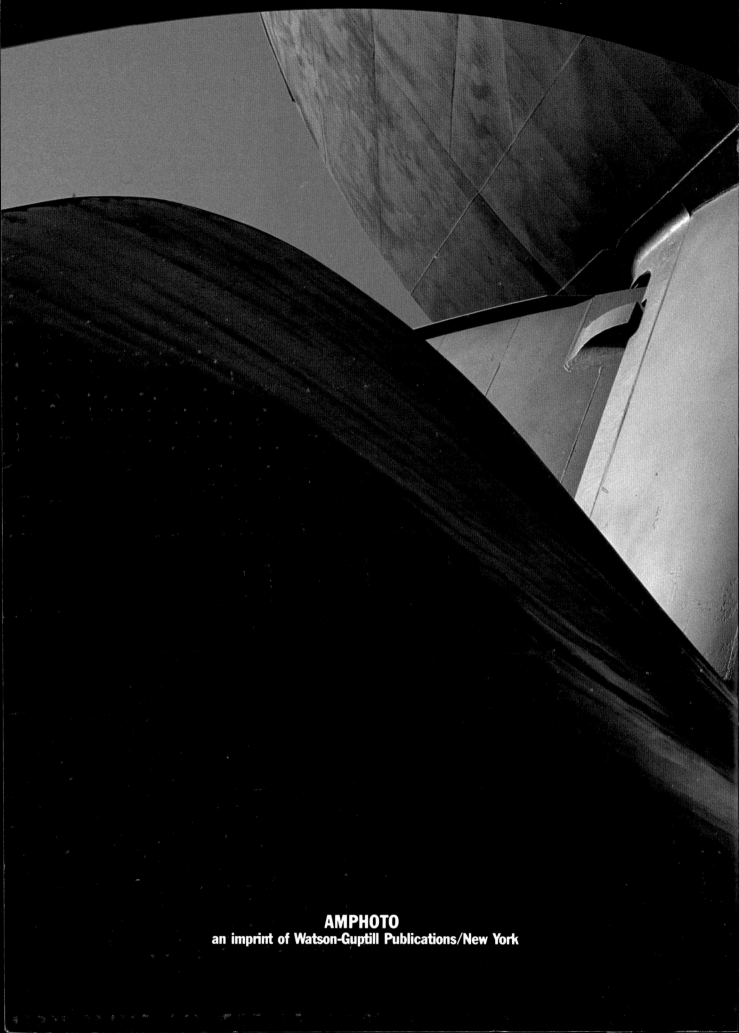

AMPHOTO
an imprint of Watson-Guptill Publications/New York

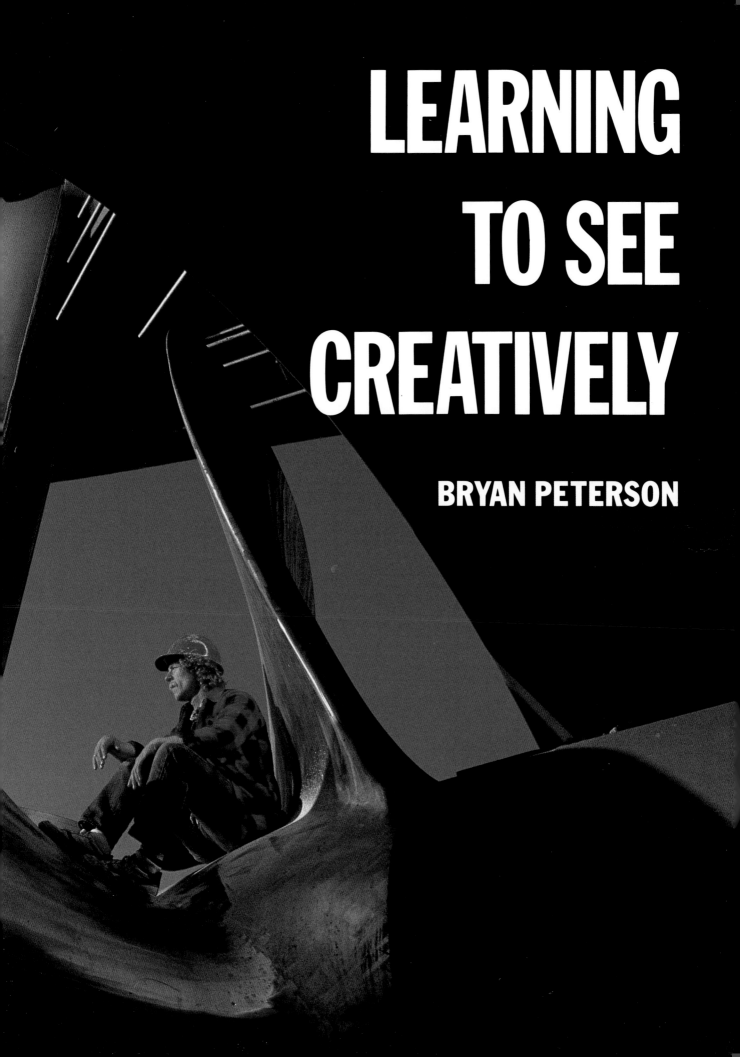

LEARNING TO SEE CREATIVELY

BRYAN PETERSON

Bryan Peterson is a professional photographer who specializes in corporate and industrial annual reports. His popular photography column appears in *This Week*, the weekly Portland, Oregon newspaper, and his photography seminars have brought his unique teaching methods to over five thousand students. Peterson's work has appeared in numerous magazines, including *Popular Photography, SLR, Pacific Northwest, Oregon, Wine Country*, and various in-flight magazines. He has received awards from the New York Art Directors' Club, the Phoenix Art Directors' Club, *Northwest* magazine, *Communication Arts* magazine, Minolta Corp., and Nikon, Inc. His clients include: Amoco; the Army Corps of Engineers; Burlington Industries; Horizon Airlines; Manufacturers Hanover Corp.; Minolta Corp.; Nike, Inc.; Nikon; Pacific Telecom; Piedmont Airlines; Skies West, Inc.; Transamerica Corp.; US Fish and Wildlife; and Weyerhauser Corp.

Copyright © 1988 by Bryan F. Peterson

First published 1988 in New York by AMPHOTO,
an imprint of Watson-Guptill Publications,
a division of Billboard Publications, Inc.,
1515 Broadway, New York, NY 10036

Library of Congress Cataloging in Publication Data
Peterson, Bryan F.
  Learning to see creatively / by Bryan F. Peterson.
    p. cm.
  Includes index.
  ISBN 0-8174-4176-X ISBN 0-8174-4177-8 (pbk.)
  1. Composition (Photography) 2. Photography, Artistic.
I. Title.
TR179.P47 1988
770'.1—dc19   87-35414
                                            CIP

Manufactured in Japan

5 6 7 8 9 / 96 95

*To my wife Valerie, whose unselfish love and support makes
my work possible, and to my son Justin, whose fascination with life's
wonders continues to be a great source of inspiration for me.*

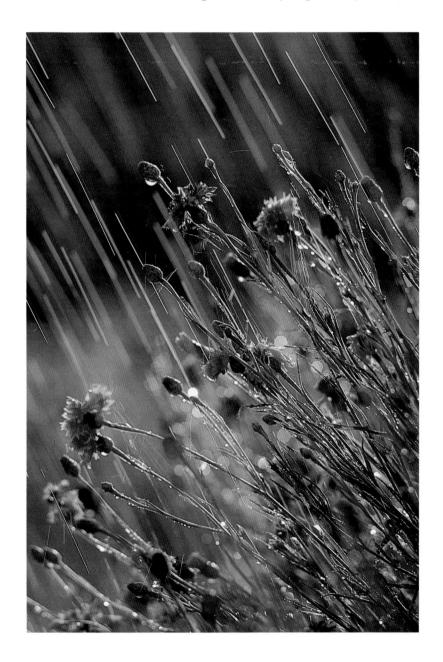

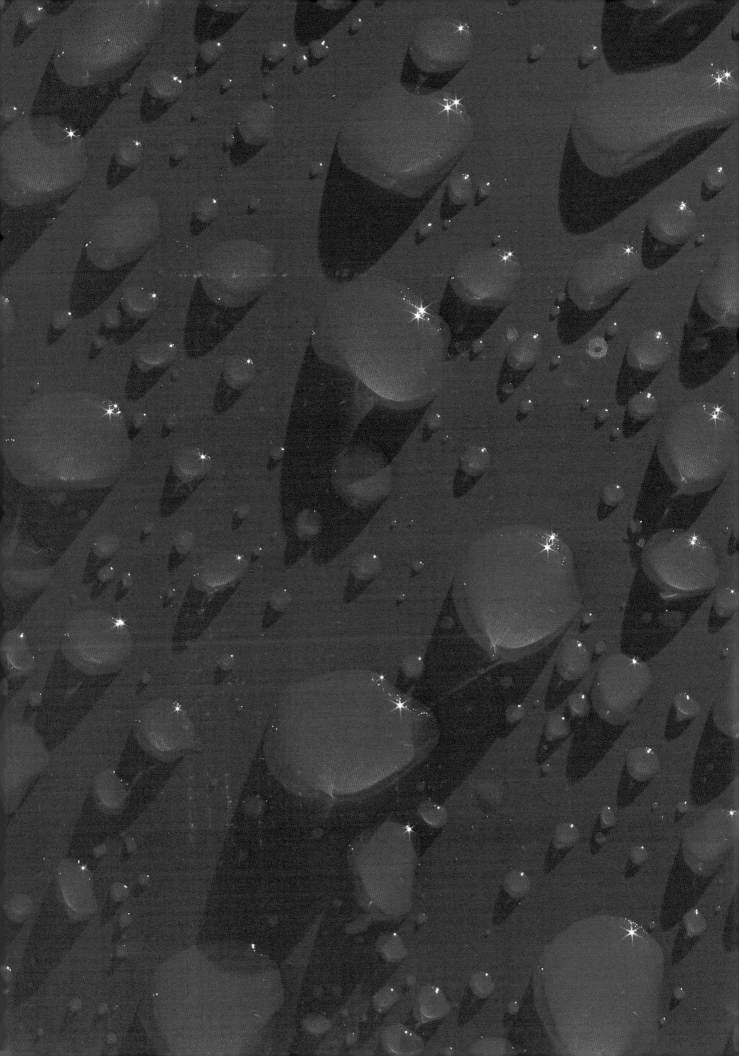

CONTENTS

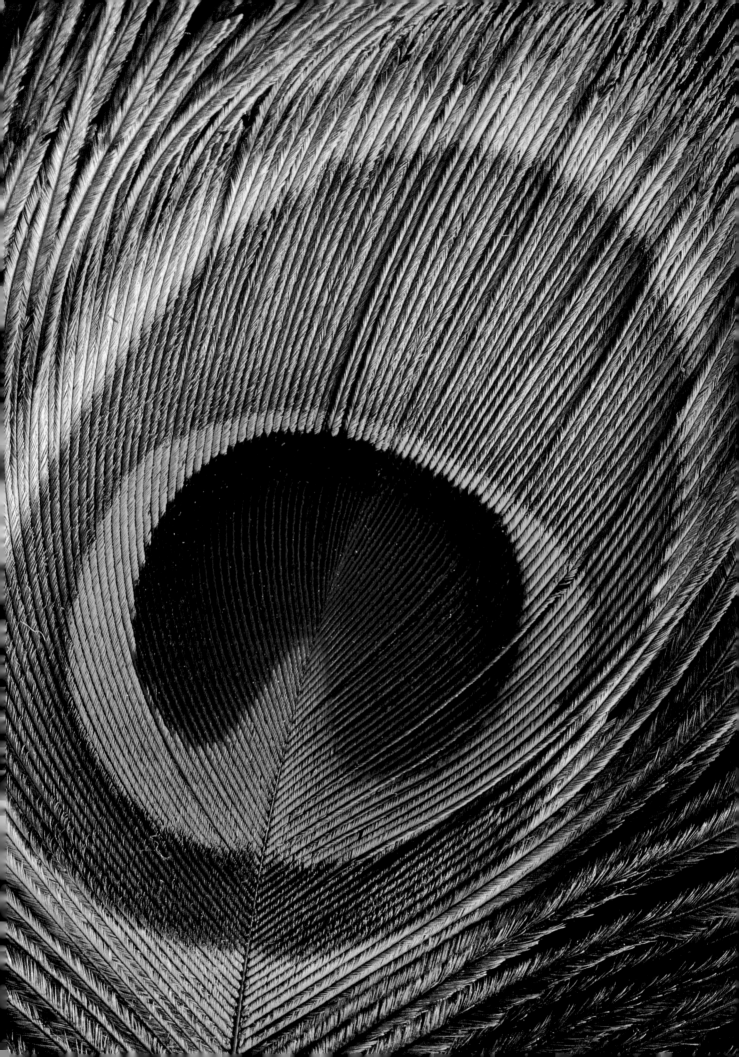

INTRODUCTION

"How can I take better pictures?" is the fundamental concern of all photographers; learning to see creatively is the answer. Of course, most of us can "see" in the ordinary sense of the word, but unless sight is guided by creative vision, picture-taking efforts seldom result in compelling imagery. To really see creatively, you must learn to acknowledge and let go of your prejudices and preoccupations. Think back for a moment. Why were some days behind the camera more successful than others? Probably because you were more free psychologically and were totally attuned to the present. Learning to see creatively also depends on your knowledge of what the camera sees. Human vision is capable of abstracting images from the environment. The camera alone can't do this. You have to make a conscious effort to use it as a tool for presenting your vision.

The aim of this book is to teach you how to recognize and avoid the visual prejudices that lead to dull, ordinary photographs and to help you get a new angle—or angles—on your pictures. There are numerous pairs of photographs included as visual aids for learning how to abstract from larger contexts. My goal as a photographer is to compose pictures by using only those parts of a scene that are essential for expressing a mood or feeling. The pictures you see in this book are by no means intended to show a so-called "right" way to deal with any of the subjects photographed; instead, each picture simply represents the way I chose to interpret that scene at that moment. I'm sharing my ideas and experiences with you in the hope that they'll shake loose your own creative vision.

Creativity, a vital ingredient in any good photograph, may best be described as a combination of inventiveness, imagination, inspiration, and perception. Don't be misled into thinking that creativity is "something for the chosen few"—its components can be learned much the same way you learned how to tie your shoes and to dress and feed yourself. I've had great pleasure in watching literally hundreds of students, who initially claimed they couldn't see creatively, turn into visionaries behind the camera.

Study the chapter on the elements of design; afterwards, you'll understand why one shape holds more importance than another and why carefully composing a number of forms is far more effective than randomly arranging them in a photograph. Before you know it, you'll begin to see creatively, too. Pay attention to my suggestions about analyzing picture elements, their emotional messages, and the roles they play in any given scene. Repeated efforts with the exercises outlined in this book will begin to reveal your own individual style, which will boost your self-confidence and lead you to even better picture making.

Every successful photograph depends on a number of variables: lens choice, point of view, composition, light, and the time of day. Although this book is not a primer on basic camera function, I've also included a section on film, *f*-stops, and shutter speeds because they play a part in creative vision. All of these subjects are covered in simple language, one at a time, with ample illustrations and exercises. Treat this information as a jumping-off point for your own experimentation. Whether or not your subjects are compelling on film depends on how *you* respond to them, not on some magic recipe for taking good pictures. You're the one who chooses the lens and the point of view and determines a range of tones based on exposure. And you're the one who finally presses the shutter at the "decisive moment."

Some people choose photography as their medium for expression because of its immediacy and realism, others because of its artistic possibilities. However, all photographers value their work as precious frozen moments that preserve special places or occasions. Should it ever seem that you have nothing to shoot, don't blame the bad weather, poor light, or lousy subject matter. Take a look in the mirror, and try to figure out how to start seeing creatively again. I will count it as a success if, after reading this book, you find yourself making excuses to go out and shoot instead of making excuses about why you're not. As Henry David Thoreau once said, "The question is not what you look at, but what you see." Enjoy!

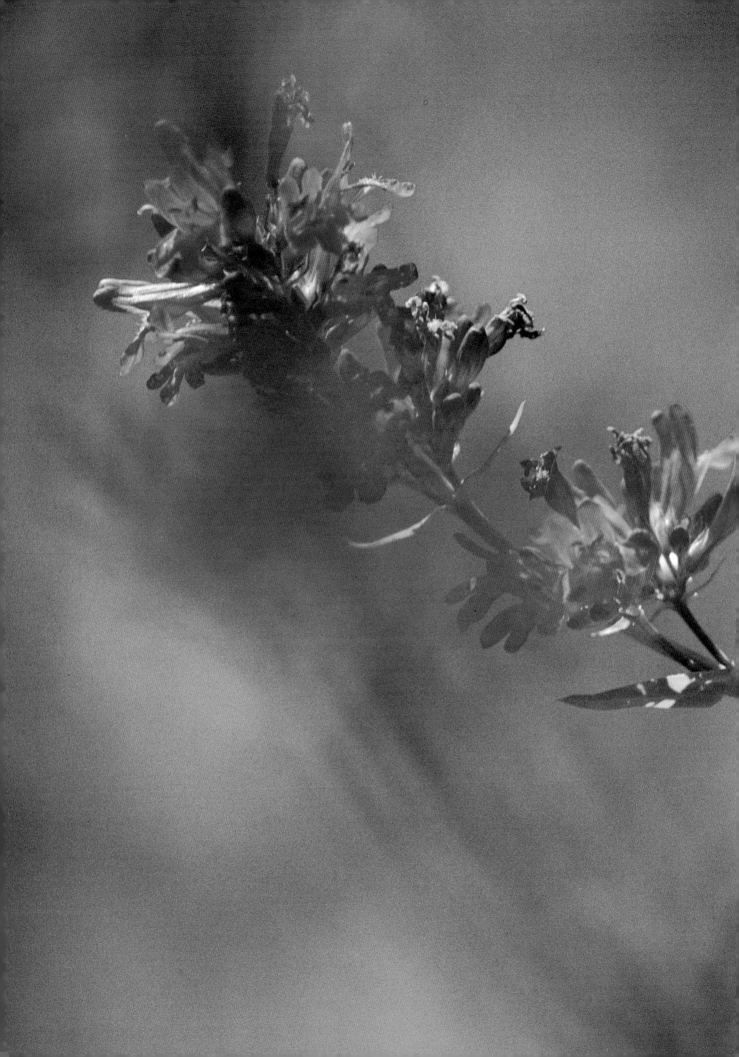

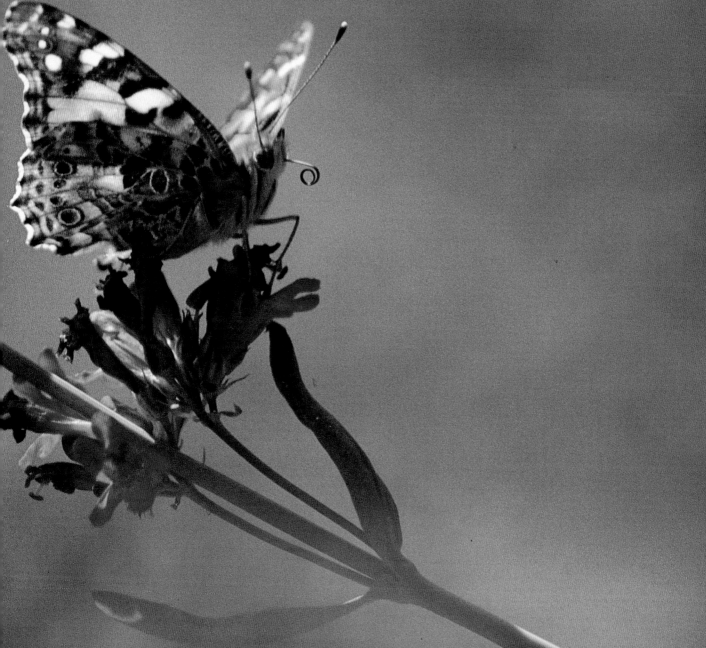

EXPANDING YOUR VISION WITH LENSES

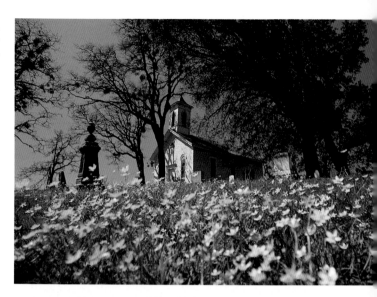

P hotography is a way to bring your imagination to life on film, but first you need to discover how your lens or lenses view the world. Many photographers are confused about the visual characteristics of the lenses they already own and carry around in their gadget bags. When you scan a landscape looking for something to shoot, don't leave your lenses in the dark; that makes as much sense as looking for buried treasure without a map. Every lens maps a unique visual path to the images hidden in the world around you. Take those lenses out of your bag, put them on your camera, and start looking.

What you see when you look through your camera's viewfinder depends on two variables: your point of view, and the focal length of your lens. Every focal length presents a different way of looking at a given subject. A standard lens approximates the angle of view familiar to the human eye. When a wide-angle lens is used from the same camera position, it reveals more of a scene and renders subjects smaller than a standard lens could. A telephoto lens does just the opposite. Rather than expanding the field of view, a telephoto zeroes in on one part of a scene, making it appear larger and closer than a standard lens could and compressing the scene's depth of field.

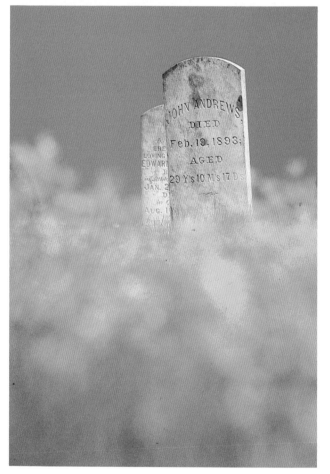

On a 35mm camera, lenses with 15–35mm focal lengths are wide angle, 45–58mm lenses are standard, and 70–500mm and longer lenses are telephoto. Zoom lenses incorporate many focal lengths in a single design, thus allowing you to change the image's magnification without switching lenses or moving closer to the subject. In addition, most zooms manufactured today include a macro feature that permits close focusing. Because the macro feature on most zooms doesn't increase magnification beyond one-quarter life-size, zooms are not considered true macro lenses.

The marketplace is currently glutted with zoom lenses. From 24–50mm wide-angle zooms, to all-purpose 35–70mm zooms and 60–300mm telephotos, each zoom promises to be *the* lens to make picture taking easier. If easier is defined as less weight in the gadget bag, I agree. But if easier is defined as greater creativity, forget it. I don't believe for one minute that any lens is going to make anyone a better photographer. That is like suggesting that Frank Lloyd Wright was a great architect because of his pens and pencils or that Claude Monet was a great painter because of his paints and brushes. The camera and the lens are simply tools that allow you to record your imagination on film. If you can't envision anything to point a standard lens at, what good will ten other lenses be?

In my early years as an amateur photographer, I ran all over the countryside with nothing more than a standard lens hooked up to my brother's Nikon F camera. This taught me the values of walking closer to a subject and of changing my point of view by

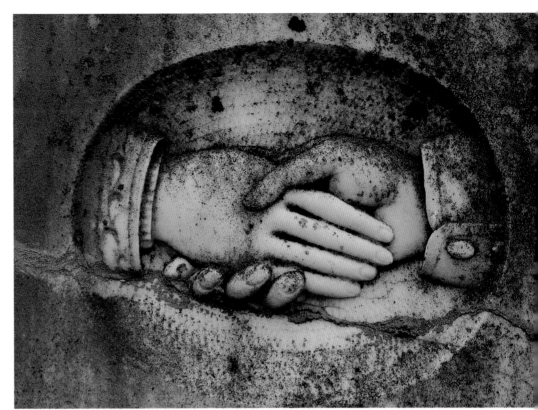

Spring Valley Community Church—it occurred to me that the name couldn't be more appropriate as I headed my car up the church's dirt driveway one lovely day in May. Following a brief walk around the grounds, I was filled with anticipation and excitement. ◆ My first choice was to do a landscape of the church and its surroundings. With my 24mm lens I got down on the ground and asked myself, "If these flowers had eyes, what would they see?"

◆ Lying there on my belly for a minute, I looked around and spotted a lone tombstone up on a small knoll. With the aid of my 200mm lens I isolated the tombstone and with a large lens opening turned the flowers into an out-of-focus yellow frame.

◆ Over the next hour I shot a lot of tombstone art with my 50mm lens, including these two clasped hands. I already felt a great deal of satisfaction, but before leaving, I took one last walk around the church. ◆ With my 24mm lens on the camera, looking up, looking down, in close, and backing away, I came upon the edge of one of the church windows. The 24mm's sweeping vision enabled me to compose the picture of the window so that it included the reflection of a nearby oak.

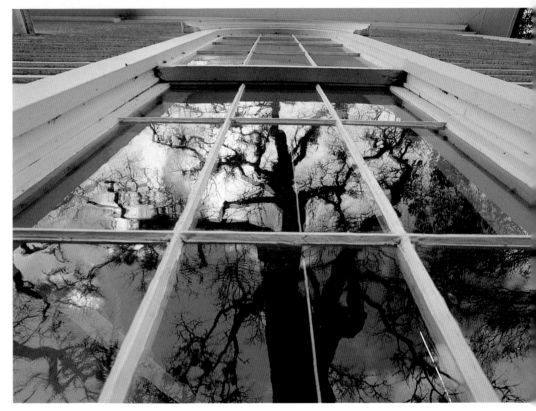

I find it helpful to challenge myself repeatedly and am always searching for fresh perspectives. The day I took these pictures was no exception. Heading out with only my 50mm lens forced me to make the most of its vision. I may have had only one angle of view, but my choices in altering my point of view were unlimited. ◆ From the road I saw a brightly painted radio tower; overhead the skies were blue. I wanted to see what my 50mm

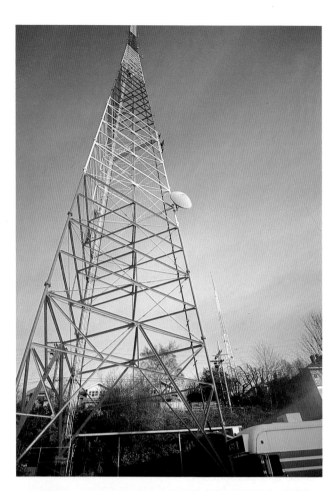

lens would see if I were to get directly underneath and shoot straight up.
◆ The photograph below clearly shows the value of putting a 50mm lens to work. Because its angle of view is greater, my 24mm lens would have recorded too much extraneous material outside the tower's perimeter. And had I shot with the narrow-angled view of my 200mm lens, the tower's depth and my perspective would have been diminished considerably.

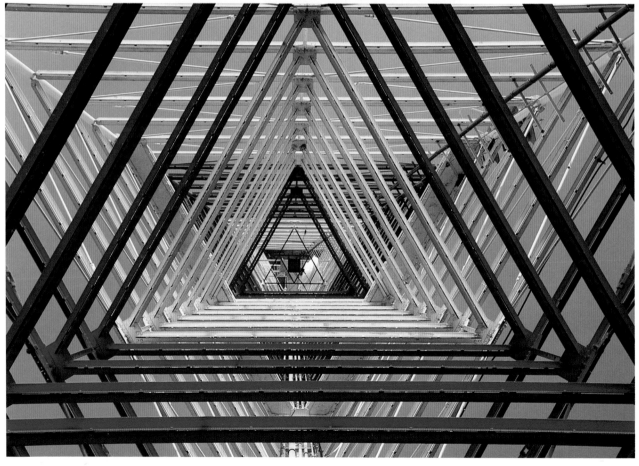

getting down low or climbing up high. It wasn't long before I knew every nook and cranny of my 50mm lens' vision. I knew its extremes, as well as its limitations; its vision was limited solely by my imagination.

A year and a half later, I plunked down several hundred dollars, purchased a 200mm lens and immediately set off on a new visual course. The space in my new images became compressed. The angles of view diminished along with the depth of field. I learned about selective focus, and perhaps the best part was discovering that distant objects now seemed a lot closer. My affair with the 200mm lens lasted for more than three months, during which my 50mm lens never saw the light of day. Shortly thereafter, the vision offered by both lenses became so much a part of me that I began seeing pictures at every turn. I used my 50mm lens primarily for landscape shots and my telephoto lens to abstract pieces out of the landscape.

Finally, almost three years later, I had the money to buy a wide-angle lens. Shock and amazement filled me as I twirled through the woods on my first outing with my 24mm wide angle. Trees bent, mushrooms loomed large in the foreground, and I was able to include distant waterfalls and the river's edge in a single frame. I soon discovered that a wide-angle lens is much like my 50mm—both are very useful for doing landscapes, but both require important material in the foreground to provide scale and perspective.

Based on my own early experiences, I've developed a photographic exercise for learning how to see called the full-immersion method. For three consecutive days I suggest you spend sunrise to sunset shooting at least five rolls of film per day. Whether you choose to do this in your own home, at the beach, in the woods, or in the city makes no difference, but you can't take more than one lens with you. The first day I'd recommend using only the 50mm, the next day your wide angle, and finally your telephoto. Those who have an assortment of lenses may experience some initial anxiety about shooting with only one lens for an entire day; however, I guarantee you'll learn a valuable lesson about looking at your subject through the lens' eye rather than your own. The goal of this exercise is to make you so familiar with each lens' vision that you become able to scan a scene and immediately select the right lenses for the many pictures springing to your mind.

Remind yourself that you can go anywhere your arms and legs will take you, and explore your subjects from unusual points of view. Avoid shooting everything at eye level; instead, squat down, climb a tree, lie on your belly, or roll over and shoot your subject framed against the sky. Walk closer to your subject and then back off from it, and observe how the background changes. When you experiment with different points of view as well as different lenses, you'll discover new ways to manipulate the fore-

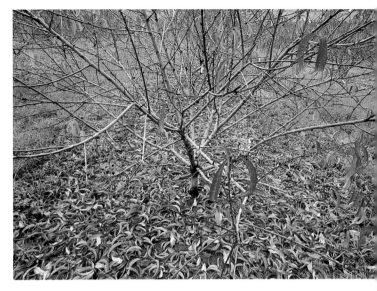

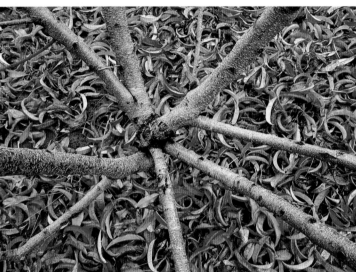

After receiving permission from the landowner, I went into this peach orchard during autumn's peak with only my 24mm lens. With the camera held up to my eye I began to walk between the rows pointing the eye of the lens up, down, and from side to side. ◆ Standing with my camera at eye level, I arched over the top of a small tree and looked down. I immediately felt as if I were seeing through the eyes of a small bird that was peering over its nest and looking down at the ground.

I had just wrapped up an assignment in Spokane, Washington. My plane, however, wasn't scheduled to leave for another five hours. I had heard about the Palouse country, an area of never ending, rolling wheat fields, and because it was nearby, I decided to investigate its photogenic appeal.

◆ After making several inquiries, I headed down the road, directions in hand, to Steptoe Butte. I'd been told that on top of the butte I could see rolling fields of wheat for miles below me on all four sides. I arrived about one hour before sunset, set my 50–300mm zoom at the 50mm focal length, and scanned the landscape. ◆ I took only a few shots, including the two you see here. To demonstrate the pulling power of the telephoto lens, I'd like you to compare the two photographs. If I hadn't been looking through the viewfinder and scanning the landscape at the zoom's 300mm focal length, I wouldn't have seen the bottom shot. Until each lens' vision has made an almost permanent impression on your own mind's eye, make it a habit to scan any given scene while looking through the camera's viewfinder.

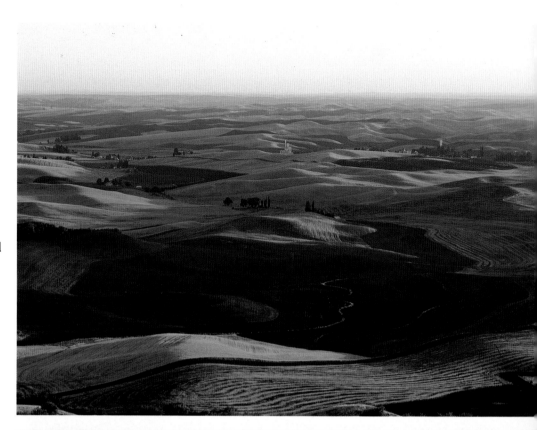

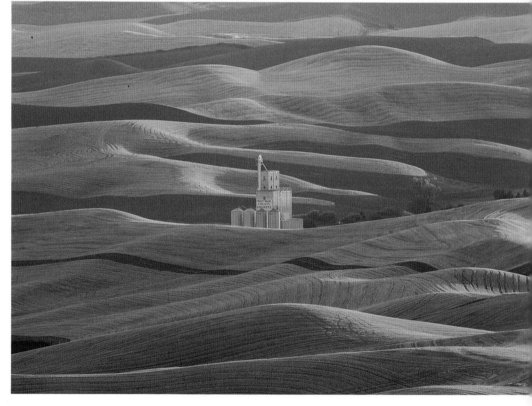

ground or change the size relationships between the objects in your pictures.

Unleash your curiosity, and allow it to soar to new perspectives. How would a seagull view the coastline from its perch? What would a mouse see as it peers up through tall grass? How does the ground below look to a squirrel as it climbs a tree? What does a dog scurrying between cowboy boots see at a rodeo? And don't overlook the perspective from an inanimate object's vantage point—how does a log in a fireplace see the living room? The choice in point of view belongs to you and your imagination, and when you compose pictures from fresh, unusual perspectives, viewers can't help but take notice.

Good photographic seeing requires an intriguing blend of experience and innocence. You have to know what your lenses are capable of seeing. Beyond that you must be willing to play with all the visual elements around you. Risking a new approach to a familiar subject may or may not succeed, but keeping an open mind and trying new approaches is the only way to make good pictures.

Because the forecast promised early morning frost, I found it difficult to sleep the night before I took these pictures. At the sound of my alarm I jumped from my bed and raced downstairs. Sure enough, a blanket of frost covered the landscape. Following a quick but nourishing breakfast, I grabbed my gear and headed out the door. ◆ I discovered that before I could unlock the car door, I needed a bucket of hot water to unthaw the frozen lock. Finally, with the door unlocked, I hopped into the car. I was ready to start the engine when right before my eyes I saw the frost on the windshield and the side window beautifully backlit by the rising sun. ◆ I took the first picture of the car with a 50mm lens so you could see the origin of the second shot that I took with my 55mm macro lens. Because depth of field is severely limited with macro lenses, I positioned the camera and tripod so that they were parallel to the car window. Focusing in very close, I exposed for the backlight. The golden light of early morning, the shimmering frost, and the added shadow from a tree branch created an interesting abstract. Over the next hour I proceeded to shoot over three 36-exposure rolls of film without leaving my driveway.

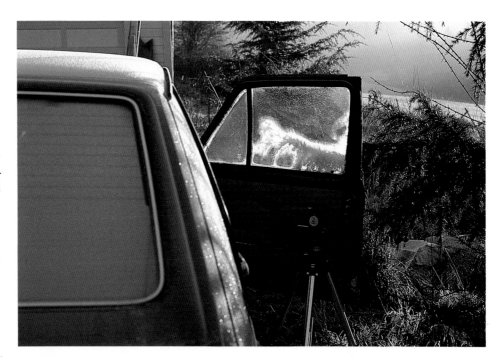

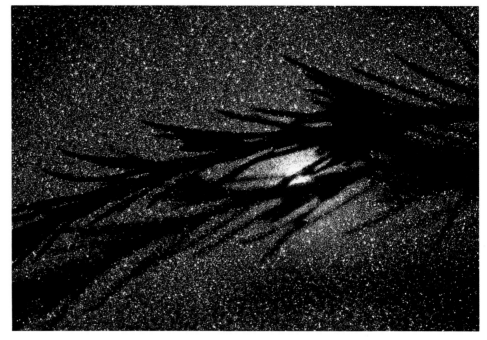

Wide-Angle Lenses

Serious landscape photographers favor the wide-angle lens because of its broad visual sweep and tremendous depth of field. But it continues to take a bad rap from some amateurs because it poses challenges for good composition. The most frequent complaint I hear is that the wide angle "gets too much stuff in the picture." That is precisely the reason these lenses are among my favorites.

I love the scope of material that wide-angle lenses bring inside the frame. Contrary to popular opinion, all that "stuff" can be fertile ground for selecting subjects to manipulate and emphasize. By carefully choosing my point of view, I have no difficulty controlling picture elements. The trick is to pay attention to the image in the viewfinder. You must learn to see everything the lens is really giving you.

In addition to pulling more objects into the frame, a wide-angle lens increases the sense of distance between them. The size of immediate foreground objects can be greatly exaggerated in relation to the background, which will increase the viewer's sense of participation; moreover, it gives you a lot of latitude in composing a picture. Although wide-angle lenses are usually associated with landscape photography, they can also render remarkable closeup images, an application you don't want to overlook. The extreme wide angles, 15–21mm, are the most susceptible to distortion and for that reason are often reserved for inanimate objects. The more moderate 24–35mm wide angles serve more general purposes. But there aren't any hard and fast rules about choosing lenses; let your imagination dictate your choice.

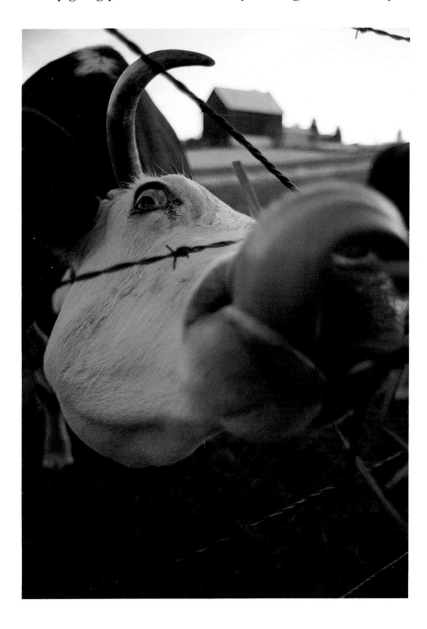

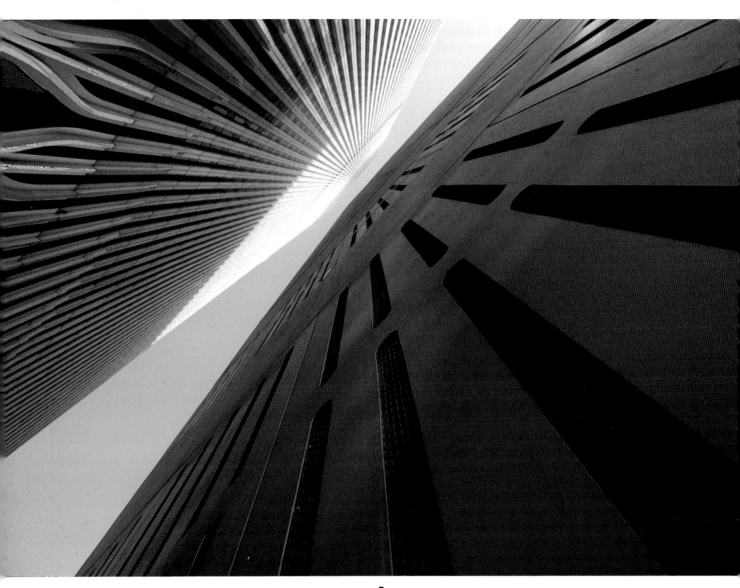

Everybody is a comedian once in a while, including this cow. Because wide-angle lenses tend to distort facial features, these lenses can turn the most mundane situation into something humorous. I spotted this cow grazing over a fence and photographed her using my 20mm lens. ◆ Wide-angle lenses are seldom used for human portraiture unless the subject is supposed to look like a caricature. You may not wish to use a wide angle to photograph your kids, but have you hugged your cow today?

I was in New York City shooting a photo assignment on lenses and perspective for *Popular Photography* magazine. I came upon this shot near the World Trade Center. With my 20mm lens and camera held up to my eye I began walking between these two buildings, looking up, moving in close on one and then the other. Rotating on my feet, I decided to compose the buildings so that they

would be on a diagonal inside the frame.
◆ The upward surge of the buildings and the deliberate diagonal framing create a tremendous feeling of movement and speed. Many photographers don't know how to cope with the tilting effect that often appears in photographs of buildings. Rather than complain about it, why not exaggerate the effect and see how you can use it creatively?

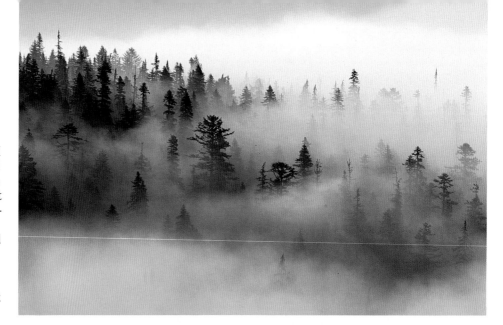

From Timberline Lodge at the foot of Mt. Hood I used my 200mm lens to shoot the early morning fog rolling through the Douglas firs. After shooting several compositions, I overheard a man, who had just driven up to the lodge that morning, talking about the dense fog at lower elevations. The way he described the fog, it sounded like pea soup. ◆ Intrigued, I hopped in my car and drove down the road, losing about 500 feet of elevation every quarter mile. When I reached the "soup," I pulled off the side of the road, grabbed my wide angle, and looked up—the towering trees seemed to go on forever. The fog and the point of view fill this composition with mystery and suspense.

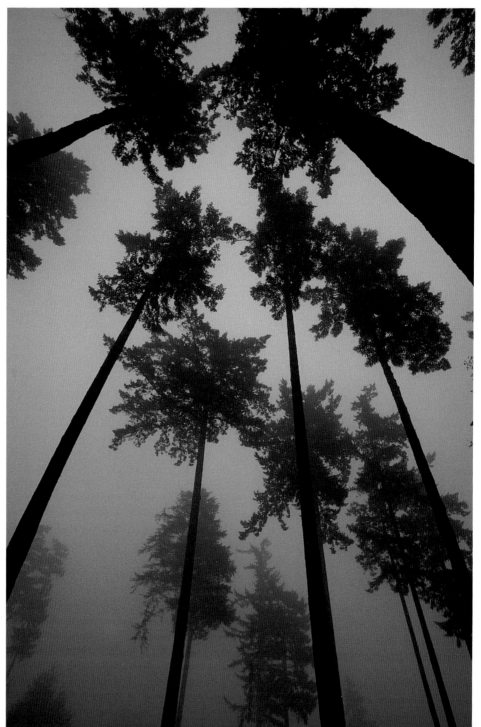

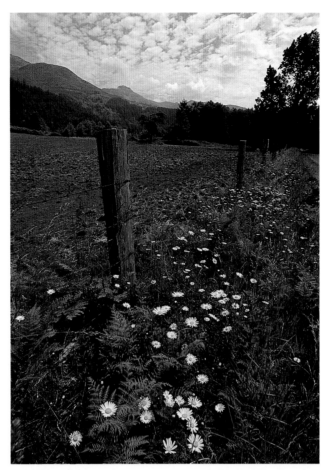

While shooting a simple landscape of roadside daisies, I heard a rustle in the grasses below my feet. Fearing the worst (I hate snakes), I jumped back onto the pavement, only to discover that the rustle was caused by a small rodent. I then became curious how the flowers might appear through the rodent's eyes. Because of the angle of view and the close focusing distance, I chose my 20mm lens to explore this ground-level perspective on the world.

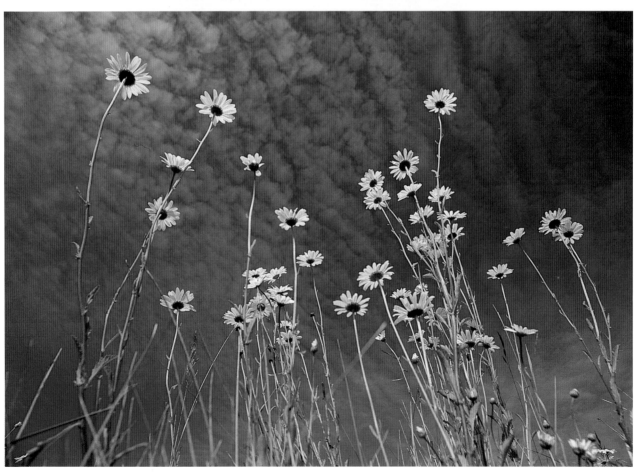

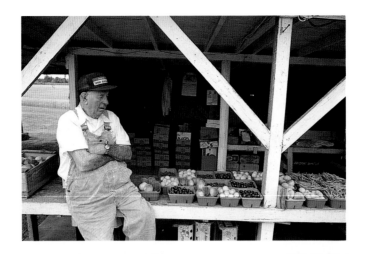

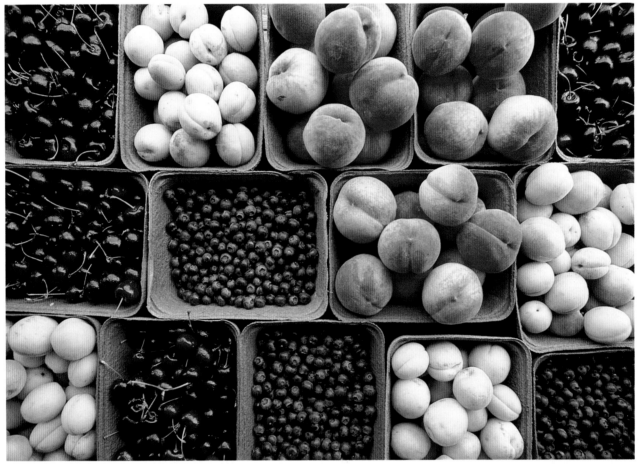

Beginning in mid-June and through early autumn, Oregon's Willamette Valley is home to many produce stands. The day I took these pictures I'd been out shooting an assignment on Oregon's winegrowers and their vineyards. Around noon I began getting hungry and drove to a nearby fruit stand. I was anxious to sample some locally grown fruit—particularly the peaches. ◆ I wasted no time in introducing myself to the farmer at the stand—making friends can really pay off in pictures. Commenting on his beautiful fruit, I asked if I could take a picture of him as well as his fruit. Reluctantly, he agreed and added somewhat whimsically, "But damned if I can figure out what you find so beautiful about my fruit." I'll be the first to admit that my portrait of him was poorly done—sometimes unwilling subjects can inhibit the best of intentions.

◆ Creating the closeup composition of the fruit was much easier since the fruit couldn't move, smirk, or talk back at me. Some photographers don't realize that most wide-angle lenses will focus as close as nine to twelve inches from the subject. At the same time, the angle of view remains the same. In this instance I used my 28mm lens and kept the camera parallel to the fruit to minimize the lens' distortion. In addition, I found that shooting straight down at the fruit on the table provided the cleanest, brightest composition.

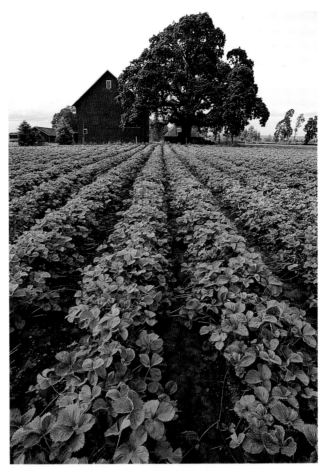

The rows of strawberries in the vertical picture form pleasing parallels that converge by the distant barn. But where are the strawberries? To find them I had to stoop down to their level. Then I asked myself, "If a strawberry had eyes, what would it see?" Laying down in the row, I focused very closely on a bunch of berries with my 20mm lens. Note that the barn in both photographs remains a point of reference for size and distance.

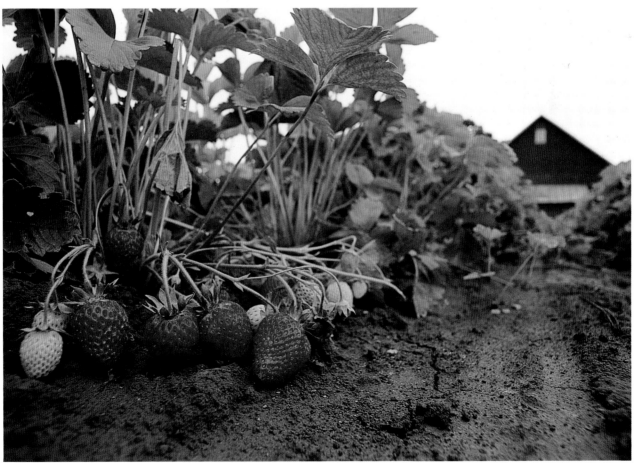

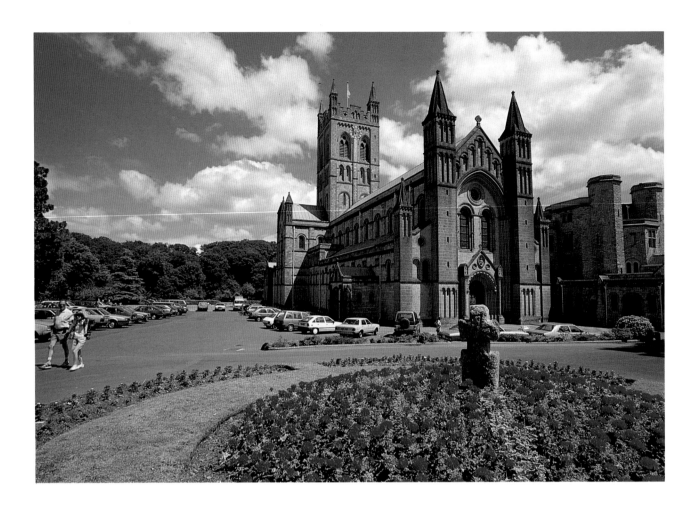

Following the road signs in Devon, England, I found the magnificent Buckfast Abbey. Unfortunately, so had a lot of tourists. Following their lead, I shot the Abbey and the flower bed filled with hot pink geraniums. And like them, I recorded everything else in my field of view, including the attractive parking lot and the couple on the left (every shot needs human interest, right?). ◆ "I didn't come six-thousand miles to take a snapshot," I silently exclaimed. To correct matters the first thing I did was to move in closer to the cathedral. Next I got down on my belly. By changing my point of view, I was able to conjure an immense foreground of flowers to block out the parking lot as well as create a picture with great depth and perspective. With my 24mm lens set at ƒ/22 and by using the hyperfocal-distance setting I was able to achieve sharpness throughout the entire scene. ◆ I've got to tell you that lying on your belly at a hot tourist spot will garner lots of strange looks; however, I remain convinced that the slight embarrassment you might experience is a small price for the emotional high of walking away with a very clean, dynamic, and unique composition.

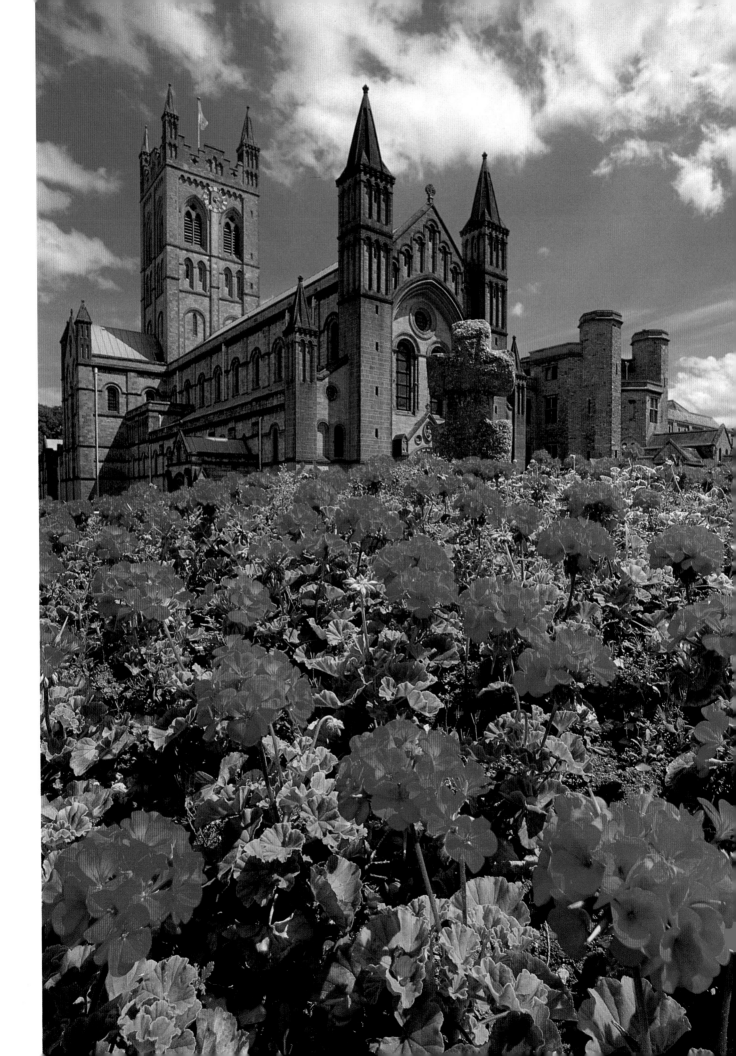

Normal Lenses

Why does the normal 45–58mm lens continue to take a bad rap? Supposedly it is because its angle of view is "so boring." Unlike the sweeping vision of the wide angle and the pulling power of the telephoto, a normal lens "just makes everything look ho-hum," or so some people think. This type of reasoning suggests that as soon as you can afford it, you should head back to your local camera shop and buy a second lens (usually a telephoto), that is, "if you're really serious about taking great pictures." I couldn't disagree more! Such logic makes about as much sense as a teenager competing at the Indianapolis 500 Motor Speedway only a week after getting a driver's license. I suggest you think of your normal lens as your learner's permit. Don't consider buying another lens until you've spent a great deal of time driving behind its angle of view.

In my case, it was an eighteen-month training period, yet within that time, I had no trouble making great pictures. Sure, it was frustrating, but that frustration propelled many visual breakthroughs. Once I had exhausted all of the obvious picture possibilities, I was forced to innovate. I soon discovered the value of walking closer to my subject, the value of changing my point of view, and the value of shooting in early morning and late evening light. Most of all, I learned to appreciate carefully composed compositions. I had no other choice!

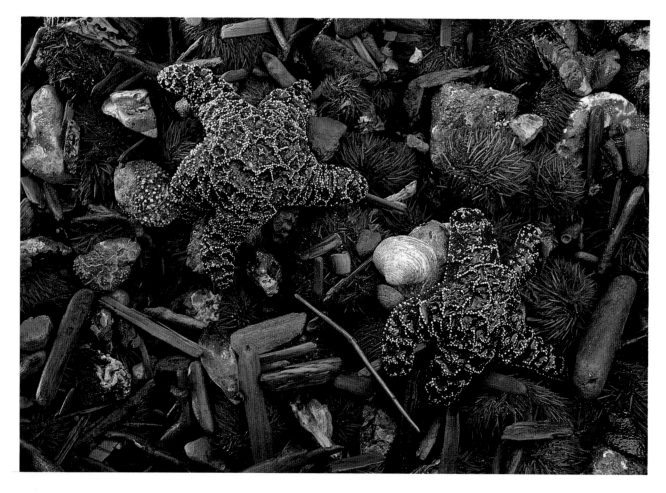

These three pictures have one thing in common— they were all taken with my 50mm normal lens. Their success doesn't rely on a lens' sweeping vision or on its pulling power, but on their careful composition. ◆ My point of view in the starfish composition was critical. By focusing my 50mm lens very closely on my subjects and pointing the camera down at them, I composed a picture in which the starfish reach out and grab the

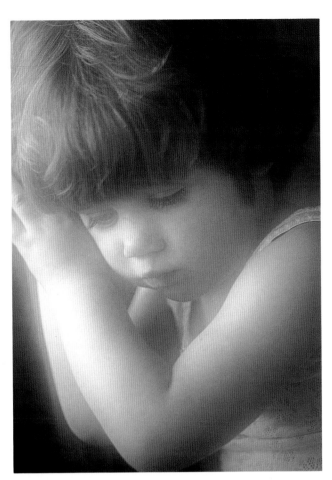

viewer's attention.
◆ Note my point of view in the portrait of the little girl. Who says you need a telephoto lens to fill the frame? With a 50mm lens you can fill the frame by simply walking closer. ◆ Limited depth of field is also possible with a 50mm lens. By selectively focusing on the foreground grass in the bottom picture, I reduced the distant barn to a supporting shape and created a strong graphic image.

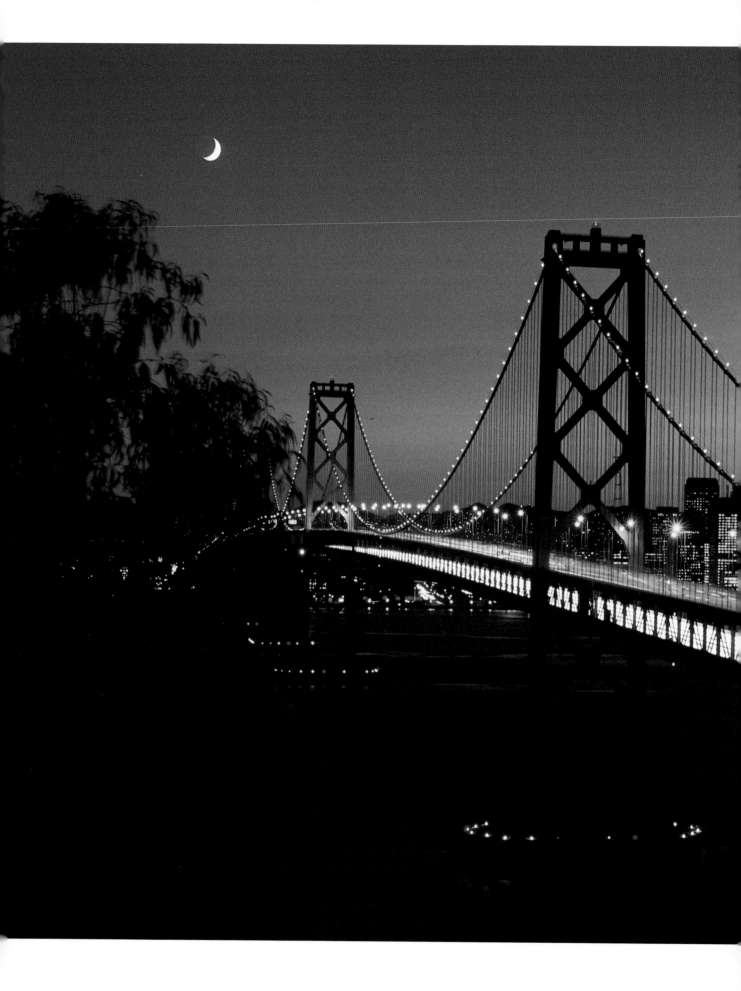

LEARNING
TO SEE
CREATIVELY

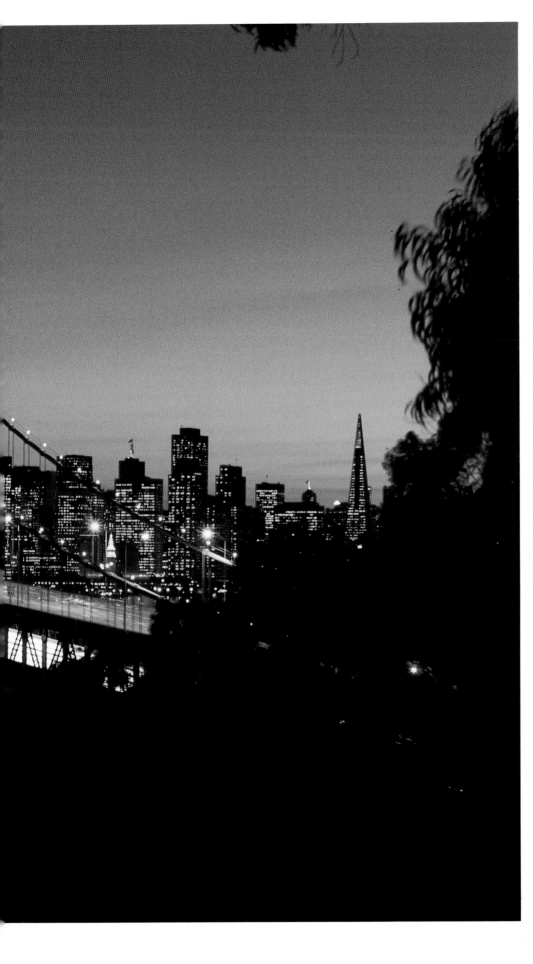

In the autumn of 1986 the Bay Bridge in San Francisco was strung with thousands of lightbulbs in preparation for its fiftieth anniversary. Several weeks before the big celebration, about a dozen photographers including me were anxious to shoot a nighttime image of the scene. ◆ Of the twelve photographers, only three of us had our normal lenses along in addition to our telephotos and wide angles. While we were busily firing away compositions with our 50mm lenses, the other nine cussed up a storm as they discovered that their telephoto's narrow angle of view cut off too much of the bridge and their wide angles pushed the city and the bridge too far back. ◆ After several of the disgruntled shooters looked through my viewfinder, they expressed surprise that I was using a normal lens. One of them made the oft-heard comment, "I didn't know a 50mm lens was good for anything, except maybe being a paperweight."

Telephoto Lenses

As every photographer who buys a telephoto lens soon discovers, its most obvious feature is that it can make big images of distant, inaccessible objects. Equally important is the narrow angle of view that contributes to the telephoto's ability to cut though visual clutter and make a subject "shout" at the viewer. Whereas a wide-angle lens is good for documenting all the picture elements in front of the camera, a telephoto reaches into that same scene and renders the details with eye-stopping clarity.

Zoom telephotos are enjoying an increasing popularity because they are ideal for portraiture, candid shots of kids at play, local sporting events, and even wildlife at the zoo. Due to major advances in lens design, many of these lenses offer exceptional sharpness. In addition, many zoom telephotos offer a macro feature that allows you to shoot closeups of such subjects as the proverbial bee on the flower.

Until recently, most telephoto zooms were either 70–210mm or 80–200mm; however, several manufacturers have now introduced 60–300mm lenses. Personally, I applaud the move because I believe the range between 200mm and 300mm multiplies a photographer's shooting opportunities tenfold. Although the size of all the telephoto zooms in this range is moderate, in many instances using a tripod is still necessary. I suggest you subscribe to the rule that says never to handhold a lens at a shutter speed slower than the lens' focal length. For example, if you're using a 200mm lens, it is a safe bet that your hand-held images will be sharp as long as the shutter speed does not fall below 1/250 second. (With a telephoto zoom you must always figure the focal length to be at its maximum—200mm, 210mm, or 300mm— even though you may be working at a shorter focal length since the overall length and weight of the lens

never changes.) When shutter speeds fall below the recommended speed for hand-holding, a monopod or firm support may suffice. If you're lying on your belly, a small bean-bag pouch or a firm pair of elbows work equally well. However, a tripod is really the best support for getting top image quality in your pictures.

Two of the unique qualities of the telephoto are its inherently shallow depth of field and its ability to compress the relative position of objects in a scene, thereby giving the impression of it being a crowded space. You'll notice that if you frame a given subject with a zoom lens at a shorter focal length, the resulting background is far more discernible than when the same subject is framed in exact proportion at the longest focal length. This lack of depth of field at the longer end is why experienced photographers choose the telephoto range for selectively focusing subjects. Combining a large lens opening with a point of view that allows them to focus through foreground matter assures them of recording out-of-focus shapes, colors, or tones around the focused object. This is a very powerful compositional technique that calls even greater attention to the focused subject. In addition, the telephoto's ability to compress space, or "stacking" as I call it, is wonderfully useful. The telephoto not only brings objects closer to you, it also jams them together.

Super telephotos range in size from 400–2000mm and are seldom used by the amateur photographer, not because they aren't fun to work with, but because of their exorbitant cost. One camera manufacturer sells its 400mm F3.5 lens for $2700; its 600mm F4 is almost twice as much! Any takers out there? Obviously, these lenses are useful, but they are reserved, for the most part, for the professional photographer, especially the sports or wildlife specialist.

I made the top photograph of a sunrise over Mt. Hood with my 28mm wide-angle lens. The sunrise is so small and at such a distance in relation to the camera that it is lost in the wide field of view. The trees, telephone pole, and road dominate this composition, not the sunrise.
◆ The bottom shot, made with my 50–300mm zoom at the 300mm setting, focuses attention strictly on the mountain, the sky, and the rising sun. Telephoto lenses are often used to photograph sunsets or sunrises because they make the sun bigger by pulling it closer to the viewer. The sky's vibrant colors and the sun symbolize unity, wholeness, and warmth, which elicits a positive viewer response.

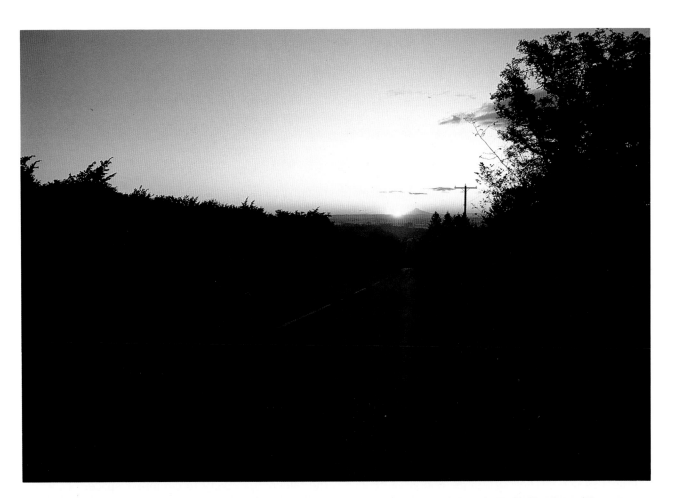

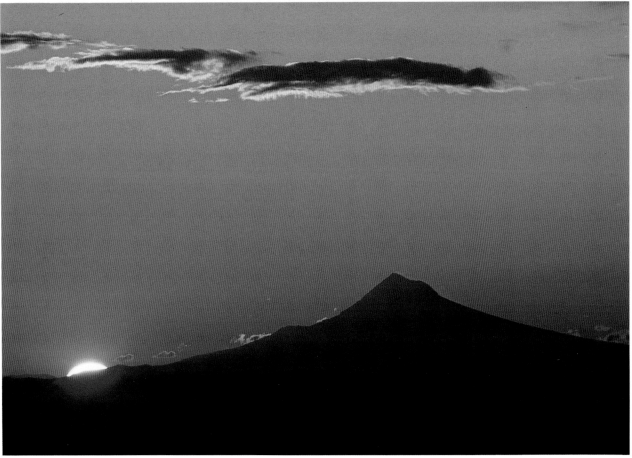

On an assignment in New York City I had just wrapped up shooting a sunset in Battery Park when my assistant shouted at me, "Bryan, check out the moonrise over Brooklyn." Setting my 50–300mm zoom at a focal length of 300mm, I made the bottom picture by framing the moon within the city. Since this was a frontlit exposure, I took a light reading of the sky to the left of the moon.

◆ After shooting almost a whole roll, I quickly zoomed back to the 50mm focal length and made the top picture so that I could demonstrate for you how the telephoto cuts through clutter and isolates only the necessary details.

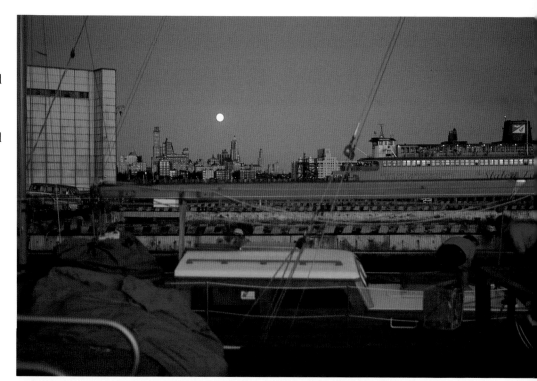

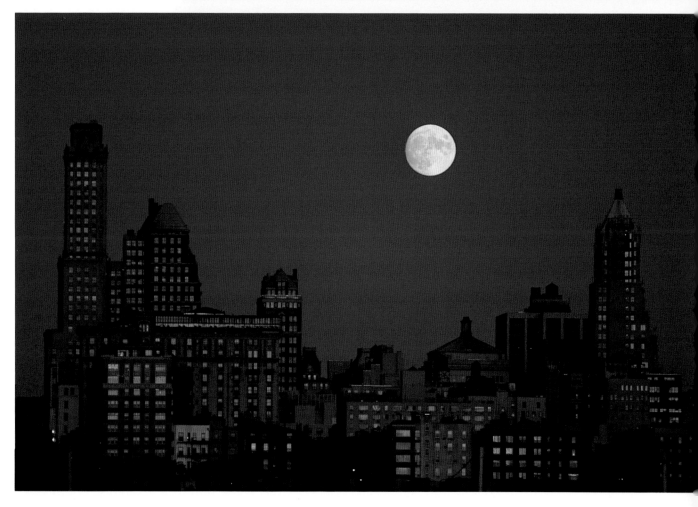

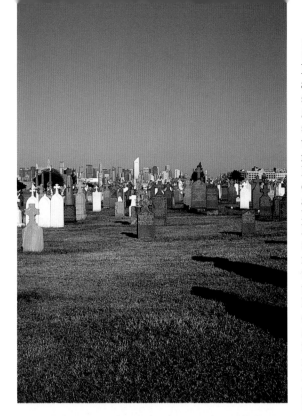

I shot these pictures in New York City to illustrate a story on lenses and perspective for *Popular Photography* magazine. Having seen Calvary cemetery in the borough of Queens many times from the Long Island Expressway, I was determined to gain access and shoot there. With the help of an assistant from New York I was driven to several locations and freely milled about the cemetery. ◆ That day I was using a 35–210mm zoom lens. To illustrate the idea of compressed space I shot the top picture at a focal length of 35mm, a moderately wide angle. Note how the wide angle pushes subjects back as if to make room for foreground interest. ◆ From the same spot I then zoomed out to 210mm to take advantage of the telephoto's pulling power and stacking effect. With my lens stopped down to f/32 I was able to get sharpness throughout the bottom image. ◆ I've had lots of fun with this photograph. Since AT&T's headquarters are in the background (the brown marbled structure with the hole at the top center of the building), I feel this would make a great tongue-in-cheek ad: "Reach out and touch someone."

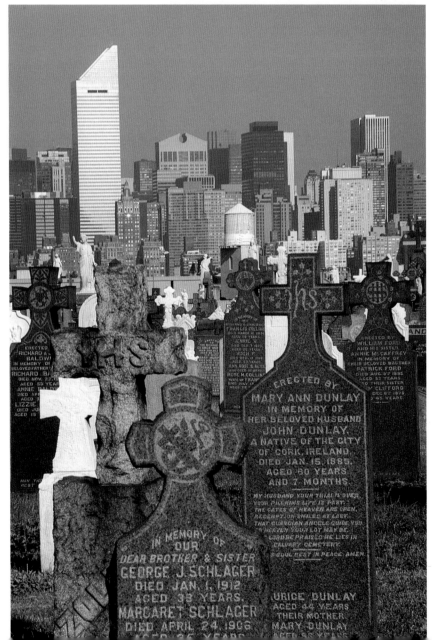

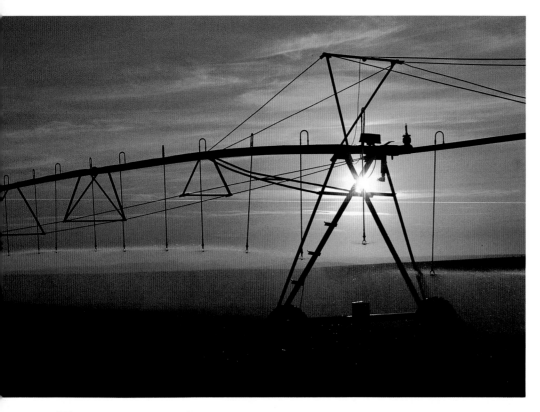

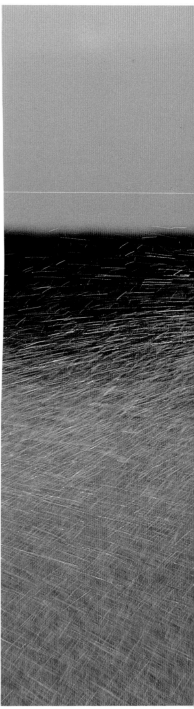

The Pacific Northwest is blessed with an abundance of water: water for drinking, water for recreation, water for hydropower, and water for agriculture. On this assignment, my job was to document a state-of-the-art irrigation system that guaranteed the farmer savings in electrical costs as well as in water usage. The theme I was illustrating was "Water, more precious than gold." ◆ It was a rather easy assignment, since I was told to make just two photographs: one backlit shot at sunset showing the whole sprinkler unit, and another detailing the gravity flow of the water. The second shot could either be backlit or sidelit; the decision was mine. ◆ Making the first shot, shown above, was easy. In fact, I was so carried away with different angles and points of view I shot almost four rolls of film in rapid succession.

However, the detail shot on the right took a bit of manipulation. ◆ With my 50–300mm zoom I was able to get a gorgeous composition of a single spigot, but the lens wouldn't focus any closer than fifteen feet away from a subject, and there I was standing ten feet from the spigot. So I used a 36mm extension tube in order to focus at ten feet and shoot the closeup of the spigot in action.

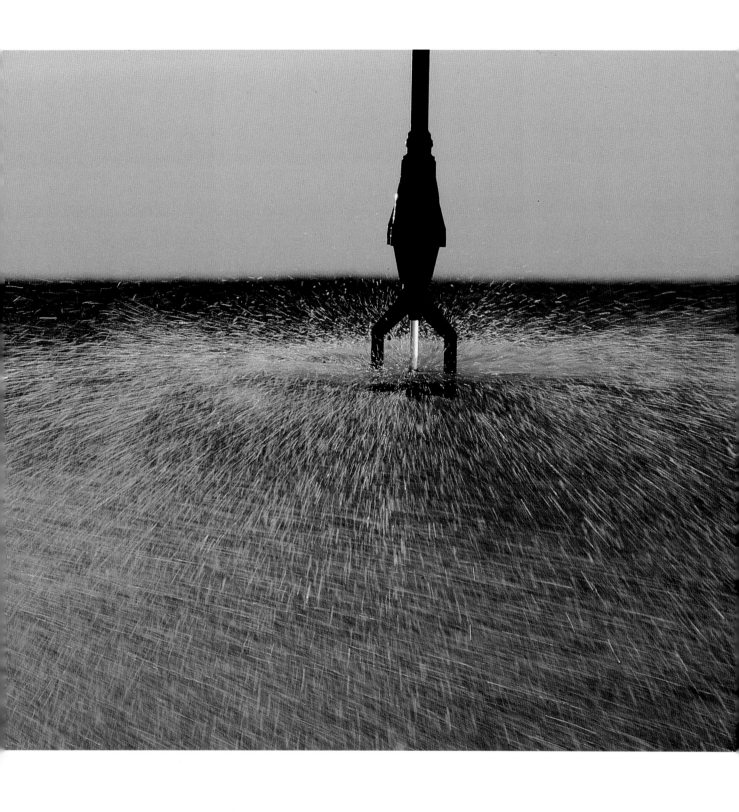

During the first few weeks of August, Mt. Adams in Washington State is a wildflower lover's paradise. On one such day I crawled about this meadow on my hands and knees framing pictures with my 24mm lens. After several exposures, I felt compelled to try some selective focusing through the sea of wildflowers all around me. Setting my 50–300mm zoom at 300mm, I began looking through the camera while focusing on flowers fifteen to twenty-five feet away.

◆ Once I discovered a pleasing composition, I set the aperture to wide open, which ensured that I would record only the subject on which I was focused and nothing else. The resulting out-of-focus spots of color in the top far right serve to strengthen the importance of my subject, the focused group of flowers.

◆ On another shooting trip in Washington State I came upon a marmot in the Olympic mountain range. A docile creature by nature, the marmot was rather easy for me to aim at and photograph, but note the point of view I chose. By getting down low, I was able to meet the marmot at its own eye level and once again selectively focus through the surrounding wildflowers.

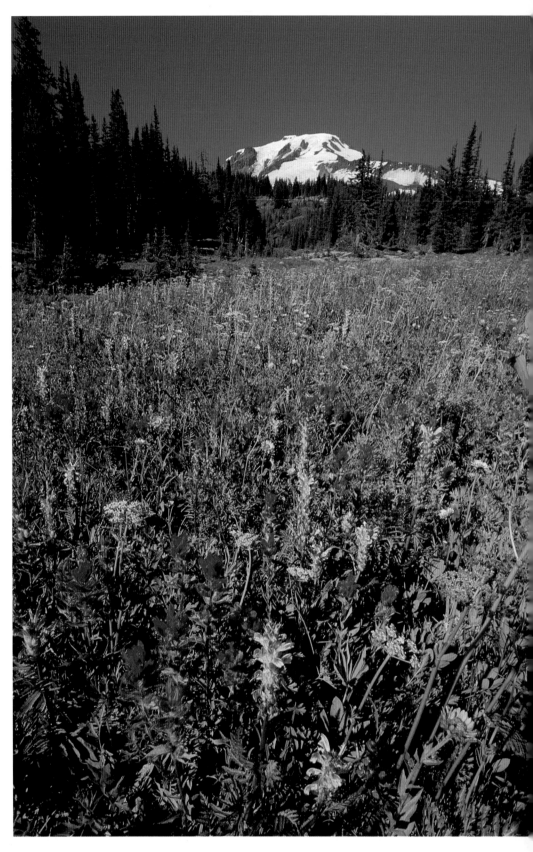

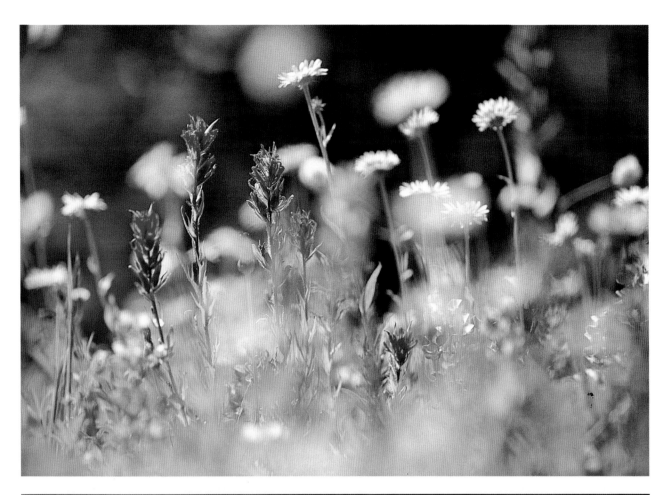

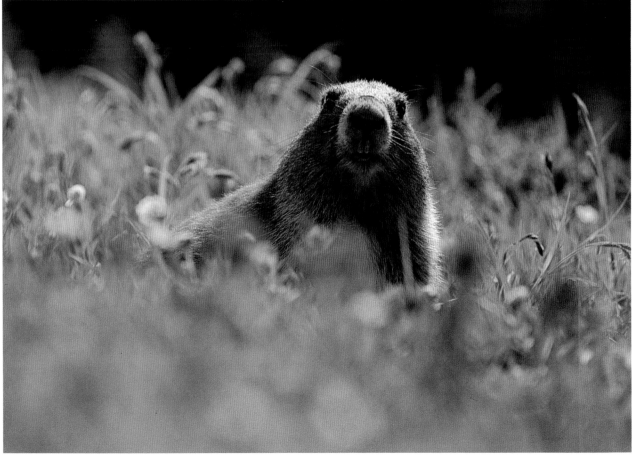

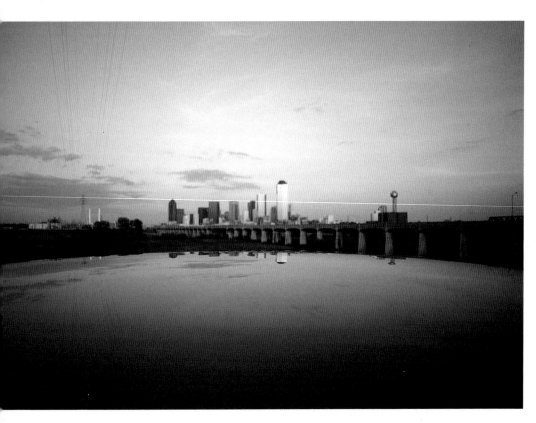

As a technique, selective focus is certainly not limited to nature. My using this technique to photograph two different cities resulted in a very similar effect in my final photographs of both places. In Dallas, Texas I was driving along a back road when I came upon a good spot for shooting the day's final light. I was intrigued with this light reflecting off the buildings in front of me as the sun set behind me. Quite by accident I spotted the skyline's reflection in the roof of my rented car (thank goodness I didn't rent a car with a vinyl top). I was curious what the city might look like if I were to shoot through the roof of the car and focus on the distant skyline. Using my 105mm lens, I composed the scene with the bottom quarter of my lens just below the car roof. With the

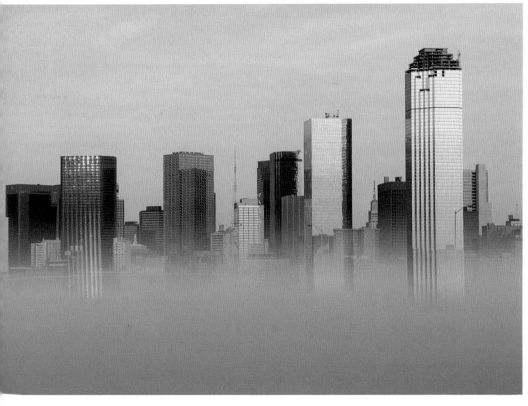

aperture left wide open I was able to create a fog effect from the out-of-focus rooftop. And there was a bonus—because the reflection of the city and the city itself were at the same focused distance, I was able to record a mirroring effect, too.

◆ Only a month later, I was in Seattle. Several days of rain had filled this large pothole near Alki Point with water. Not wasting a beat, I lay down at the edge of the puddle with my 105mm lens. Keeping the aperture wide open, I focused through the puddle to the distant skyline. Once again, I was able to record a mirroring effect and throw the puddle out of focus. Seattle residents give this photograph several double takes since at first glance it appears that Puget Sound was experiencing an abnormally calm day.

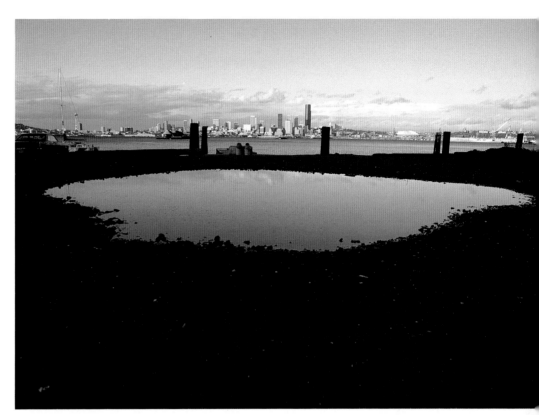

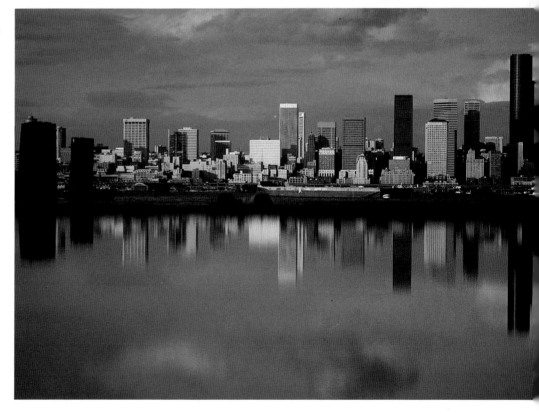

Macro and Closeup Lenses

Sooner or later, most photographers develop a craving to see the world from a closeup point of view. The camera industry accommodates this desire by manufacturing a multitude of different focal-length zoom lenses—most of which include a macro, or close-focus, feature—as well as closeup filters, macro-converters, extension tubes and true macro lenses. All this equipment is designed to allow photographers to explore the many microcosms everpresent within our larger world. Sometimes these visual journeys carry a photographer so close to a subject that reality fades away and a world of geometric elements emerges.

Because closeup photography offers so many possibilities for composition, such work dispels the photographer's common complaint that "there was nothing to shoot today." An ant foraging for food provides an apt metaphor. Daily, the ant ventures out of its hole in search of sustenance. When it returns, its pincers are filled although it rarely travels much farther than fifty feet. A photographer covering the same ground with a closeup lens could also return home laden with spoils from the hunt. The world is a very big place for the closeup lens as well as the ant.

Closeup photography involves a lot of unusual camera positions, such as knee and belly points of view, particularly when you're shooting nature subjects outdoors. An added complication is that the depth of field is very shallow at close-focusing distances, even at an aperture of $f/22$. The only way to compensate for this limited range of sharp focus is to keep the film plane parallel to the subject whenever possible, thus ensuring the sharpest possible image. In addition to steadying the camera, using a tripod can make paralleling closeup subjects much easier.

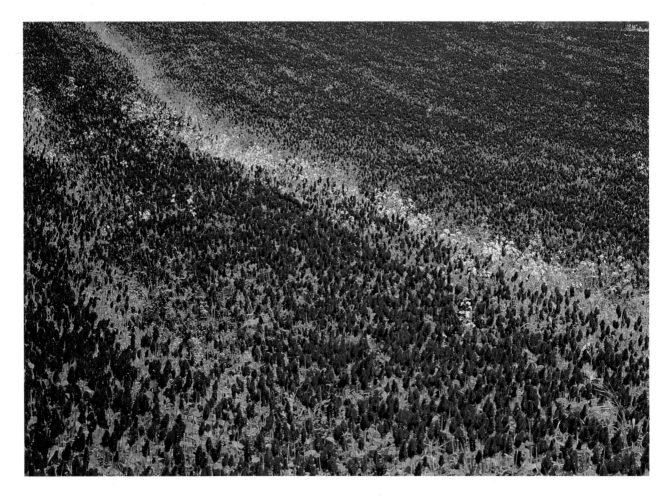

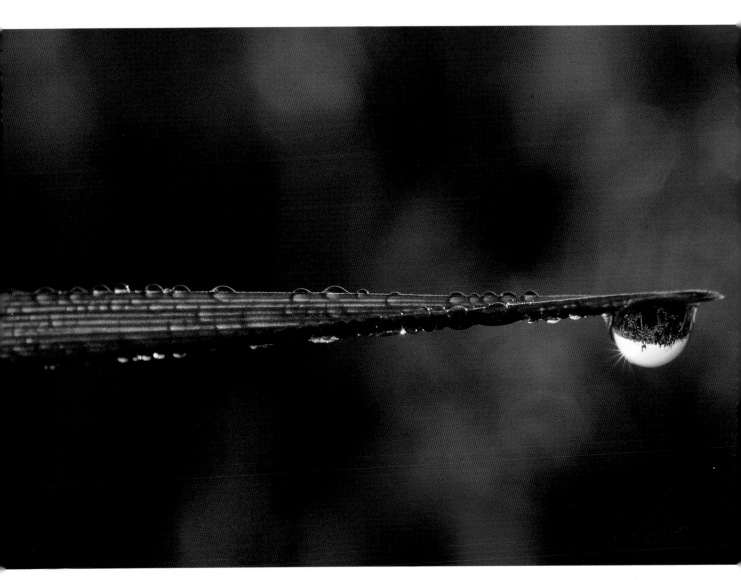

Nature continues to be the favorite subject of closeup photographers. It offers such an abundance of closeup subjects—flowers, seed pods, mushrooms, leaves, feathers, sand patterns, tree bark, and frost to name just a few—that its popularity should come as no surprise. My personal favorites are dew-laden spider webs and grasses, both of which require absolutely still air to photograph, a prerequisite that at times can challenge your patience. ◆ One morning I was out shooting the crimson clover fields that during May carpet the landscape around my neighborhood. After a few quick shots with my 105mm lens, I switched to my 55mm macro lens and began investigating the droplets of water from the previous night's rain hanging on the blades of grass. ◆ Several minutes later, I came upon a perfect subject. Adding a 36mm extension tube allowed me to make this extremely closeup shot. Keeping the subject parallel to the film plane and with my aperture stopped down all the way to ƒ/16, I was able to record the image with exacting sharpness. Note how the dew drop contains its own fisheye image of the surrounding landscape. If you turn the picture upside down, the microcosm in its reflection is much more apparent.

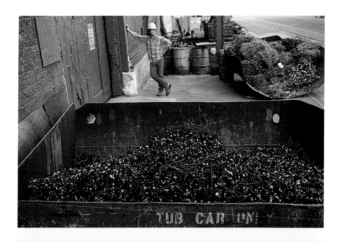

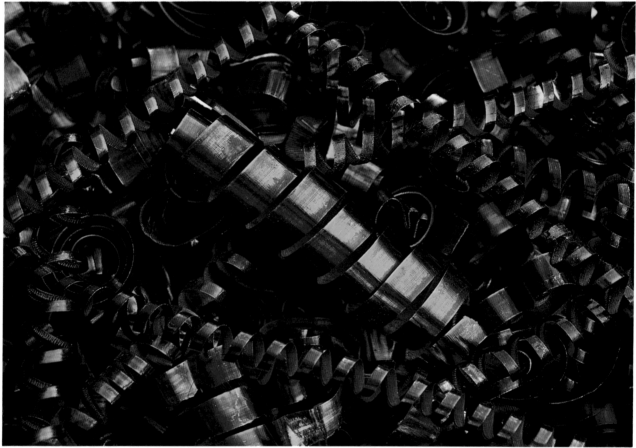

Opportunities for closeup work are just as abundant in junkyards, schoolyards, and even city dumps as they are in nature. Have you ever looked for closeups in industrial areas? You may symbolically associate the word "industrial" with loud noises and dirty air, but if you put your prejudices aside for a day, you'll discover that industrial areas are fertile grounds for capturing abstract images. ◆ Week-ends are usually best for scouting and shooting in industrial parks since most are then running with a skeleton crew. Keep this in mind since once you're inside such an area, you may find yourself snooping around alleys and dumpsters, and the last thing you want to do is call attention to yourself. ◆ On one such Sunday I came upon a dumpster bursting with metal shavings. They were predominantly blue and purple, and I was struck by the contrast of these subtle, calm colors adorning the hard-edged metal shavings. After I had found an arrangement of shavings that I liked, I mounted my 35–70mm zoom lens and camera on my tripod. Shooting straight down in the macro mode, I set my aperture at ƒ/22 to assure uniform sharpness. ◆ I must confess I went a bit wild with this stuff. After I had made almost sixty exposures, one of the workers inside the plant came out to take a cigarette break. He gave me a hard look and said, "What the @#%&*#@ are you doing there, boy!" None of my explanations appeased him until I convinced him to take a peek through the camera to see what I found so fascinating. To make a long story short, I ended up selling him a print.

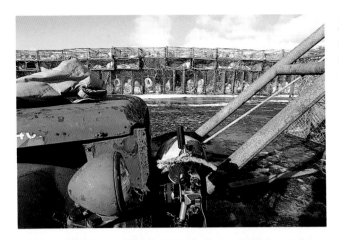

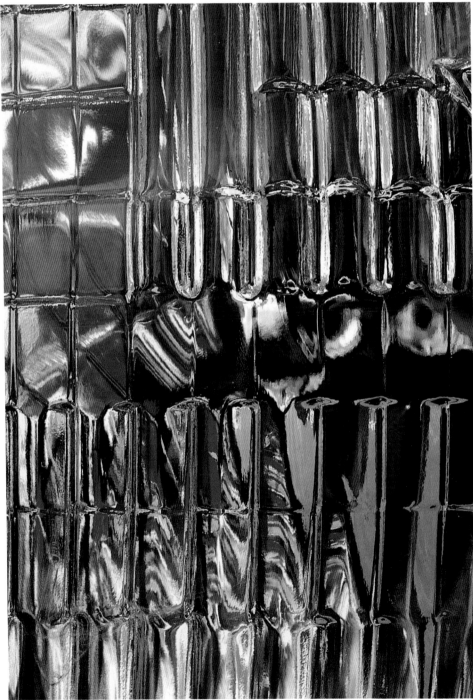

Several years ago, I was in Kodiak, Alaska shooting an assignment for a telecommunications company. One morning prior to meeting a crew of linemen, I pulled my rented car into a storeyard for crab pots. These traps are used by commercial fishermen who brave the Bering Sea during the crab season to catch giant Alaskan King crabs. What had caught my eye were all the colored buoys.

◆ Whether I was too preoccupied with the next day's shooting schedule or was just plain tired, I don't know, but I couldn't come up with a composition that held any lasting appeal. At times like this, I always reach for my macro lens. I learned long ago that it can break through any feelings of inertia—if you take the time to look through it, that is. ◆ As I ventured about the yard, I came upon several really exciting compositions, one of which was the front headlight on a rusty jeep. Reflections have always fascinated me. Any reflective surface—glass, mirrors, polished chrome, lakes, rivers, or freshly polished cars—are good sources of reflections.

◆ Studying the headlight, I noticed my red parka glinting off of it. Since it was too cold to take off my jacket and position it for the best reflection, I searched the grounds nearby and found a tattered, red plastic cup and a piece of yellow plastic rope. I set the camera and tripod up so that the film plane was parallel to the headlight and positioned the red and yellow objects on the tripod handles facing the headlight. The blue that you see came from the clear blue sky.

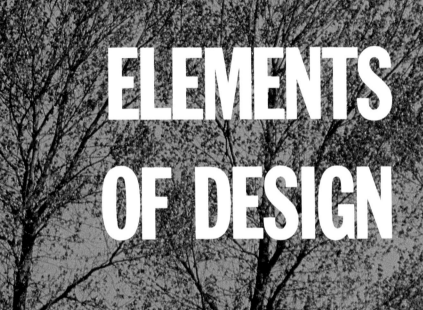

ELEMENTS
OF DESIGN

What kinds of photographs command the most attention? Usually those that involve commonplace subjects composed in the simplest way. Successful pictures are limited to a single theme or idea and are organized without clutter. These powerful compositions stand in sharp contrast to most pictures taken by amateur photographers. In their haste to record the image, many end up with pictures that have too many points of interest. The resulting confusion alienates the restless eye, motivating it to seek visual satisfaction elsewhere.

The visual elements photographers work with are line, shape, form, texture, pattern, and color. Every photograph contains at least one of these elements, regardless of the subject, and these elements have great symbolic value—particularly line, shape, and color. They can be experienced as either hard or soft, friendly or hostile, strong or weak, aggressive or passive. Most of the time you see and utilize these elements with unconscious abandon. Your memory and experiences affect your sensitivity to various visual components, and this in turn affects how you use them in your compositions.

I'd like to recommend an exercise for training your conscious mind to observe the various design elements and the way you already use them. I think you'll find the process enlightening. Let me add that I

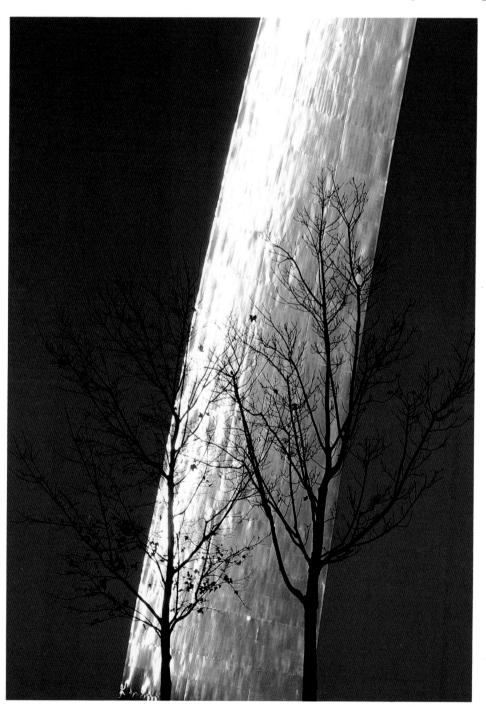

After shooting an assignment in St. Louis, I made a point of visiting its famous arch. Walking toward it, I turned a street corner and was blasted by the sunlight reflected off the arch's metal surface. With a 200mm telephoto lens I zeroed in on a piece of the arch, and by moving closer I was able to arrange two small trees in front of it.
◆ The picture's charge comes from its symbolic use of lines. The thick line of the arch carries the most visual weight and sets up a nice contrast against the thin lines of the fragile trees. There is added tension from the light glinting off the arch like a lightening bolt, or it could symbolize a rainbow and its promise of fairy-tale riches.

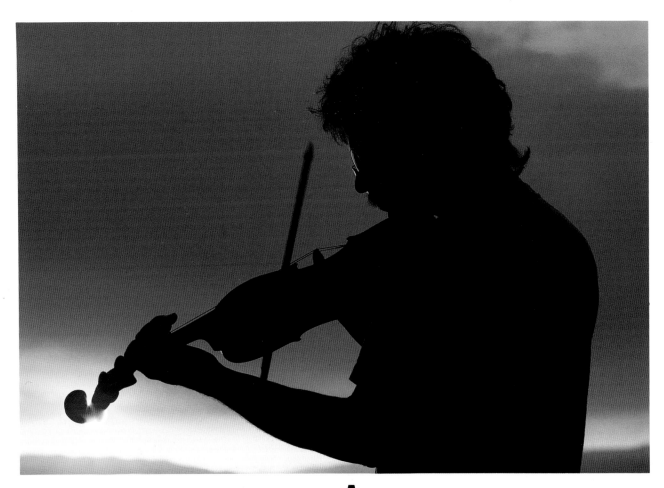

don't normally suggest exercises that concentrate on visual themes because photographers should avoid developing arid preconceptions about composition. Like having a one-track mind, focusing on only one visual element can keep you from experiencing an entire image; however, the following exercise is designed to enhance your powers of composition by acquainting you with your own visual prejudices—your strengths as well as your weaknesses.

First, gather seventy-five of your pictures, preferably without people in them. Set them aside, take a sheet of typing paper, and draw six columns on it. At the top of each column list one of the following: line, shape, form, texture, pattern, and color. Now begin looking at your pictures, one by one, with a critical eye. Carefully study each one, and make a check mark in the column that best describes the element(s) that dominate the composition. After you've looked through all seventy-five, note which columns have the most check marks. (It is likely that at least one column will have more check marks than the others.) Consciously or not, we all favor certain design elements. Both the content and arrangement of your pictures reveal something about your psyche—that is, assuming that your reason for taking pictures flows from your own feelings and responses and isn't simply an outward attempt at duplicating someone else's style.

At an outdoor concert in Oregon I photographed this musician playing in front of the setting sun. Note the power of the subject's shape, which I deliberately made into a silhouette. ◆ A silhouette is the purest shape to arouse the senses, and as the most basic form of identification, it is the most fundamental visual element. Silhouettes prevent bias; for example, seeing only the musician's shape allows you to hear bluegrass, classical, or jazz music, depending on your orientation. Like old-time radio, a silhouette frees your imagination since you have no other means of reference. Combining line, shape, and color—three of the most powerful design elements—made this a dramatic composition.

Which columns have the least check marks? Note the elements that received the lowest scores; then at the next opportunity, grab your camera and head out the door with the goal of identifying and isolating these design components. Take only a telephoto or tele-zoom lens with you. These lenses reduce perspective, which enhances good visual design since the illusion of depth has been eliminated. As discussed earlier, telephoto lenses also have a narrow angle of view that eliminates the surrounding clutter, allowing you to focus on the specific visual elements you want to emphasize.

Line

Lines are all around us, bringing direction to our lives. Some lines, such as the road to Grandma's house, lead us toward something wonderful; others, such as the road to safety, lead us away from danger. Lines evoke varied emotional responses; for example, sitting in long lines of traffic is irritating, but a long lifeline on your palm is a pleasure. Lines can symbolize wisdom and experience ("The many lines on the silver-haired man's weathered face spoke of his wisdom and experience"). A jagged line can symbolize fear ("Be careful with that broken pane of glass!"), or it can symbolize powerful energy ("Wow! Did you see the lightning storm last night?"). Curved lines represent nature, wind, water, the human body, and God's work.

The direction a line takes determines its symbolism. Horizontal lines imply tranquility and are thus considered the most stable ("From the bow of the ship to the distant horizon the ocean is calm"). Feelings of pride and dignity are reserved for vertical lines. Conventional wisdom tells you to "stand tall and firm" if you feel strongly about your convictions. Diagonal lines aren't calmly horizontal or proudly vertical but evoke feelings of movement or speed. For example, a ladder leaning against a house is a vehicle for up and down movement. Lines also have visual weight, and thick lines symbolize greater strength than thin lines. Being conscious of the hidden messages delivered by lines will allow you to manipulate a photograph's emotional impact on the viewer.

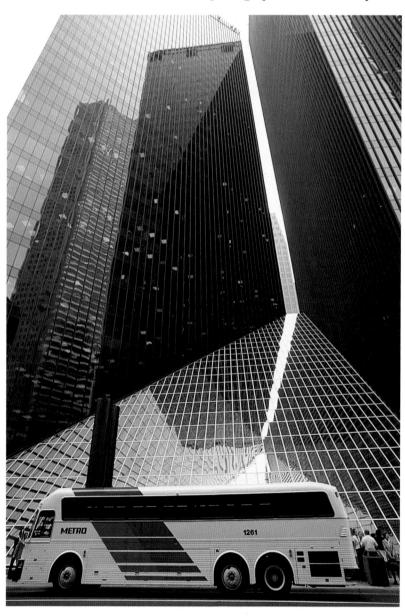

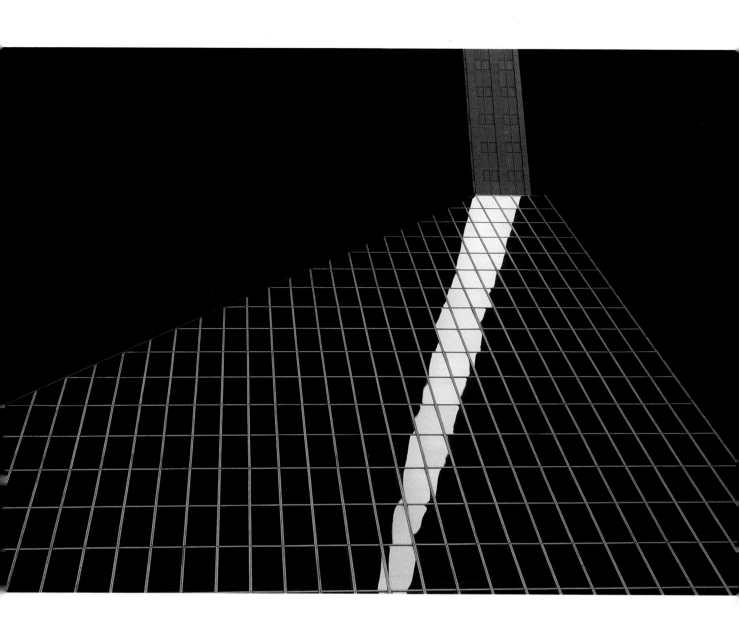

I've only been to
Houston, Texas once, but
I'll never forget it. Down-
town Houston is a treasure
chest filled with visual design elements. One after-
noon, I was working on
the street with my
35–70mm and 200mm
lenses when I was struck
by the Pennzoil Building's
multitude of lines and
shapes and the lines of the
bus below. I quickly fired
off several frames with the
35–70mm at the 35mm
focal length. ◆ Then I
decided to do a closer
study of line, so I
switched to my 200mm
and zeroed in on the white
shaft of reflected light
from the sky. Recorded in
marked contrast to the
surrounding darker tones,
this strong line reminds
me of a bolt of lightning
breaking through the night.

Along central Oregon's coast, sand dunes and trees abound. I spotted lots of lines on the side of this dune. Walking through the brush, looking every several seconds through my 200mm lens, I chose not to stop until my viewfinder was filled only with lines. Although my final picture incorporates both vertical and diagonal lines, the latter are responsible for evoking feelings of movement and speed and filling the picture with tension.

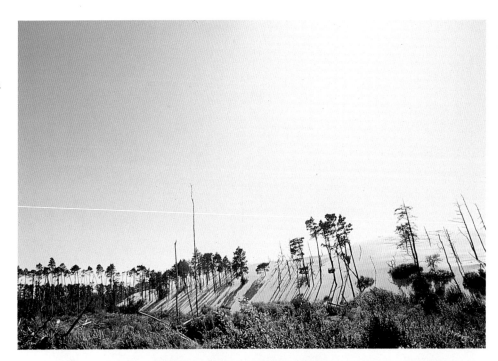

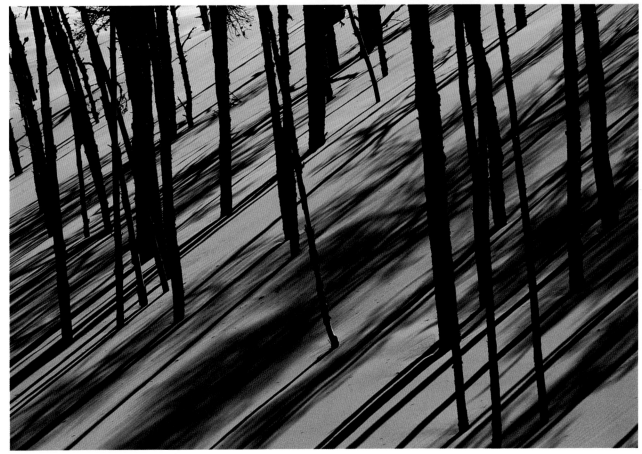

September and October are my two favorite months for shooting in roadside meadows. Early morning fills the meadows with dew, and the low-angled sun backlights the ubiquitous pods and spider webs. The yellow-flowered Scotch broom develops lots of green seed pods. When backlit, the transparent pods vibrate with energy. Although solid objects, such as people and buildings, become dark shapes when backlit, transparent objects seem

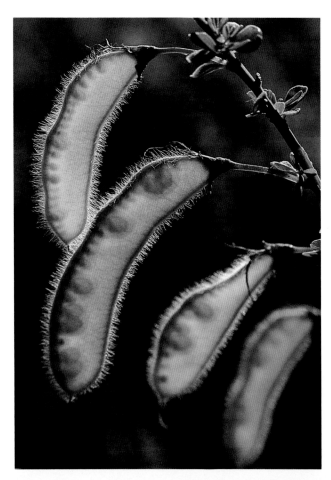

to glow. ◆ With my macro lens and several extension tubes I was able to isolate a small segment of one of the seed pods. Note how by moving in much closer—and thereby increasing the size of the broad, curved lines—I was able to give the seed pod a greater sense of weight. In addition, by deliberately tilting the camera's position on the tripod until it was in a diagonal format, I was able to create added tension in the composition.

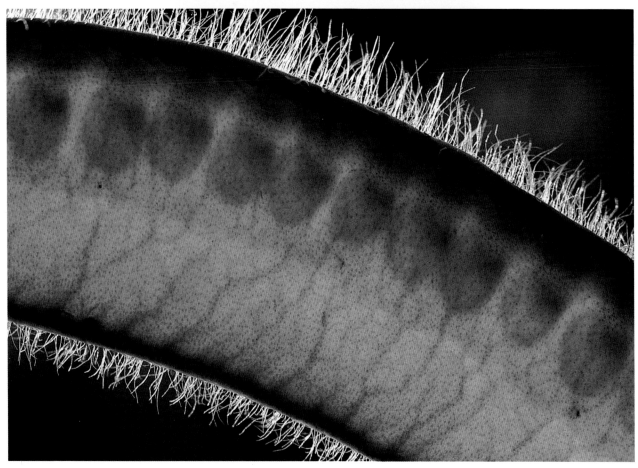

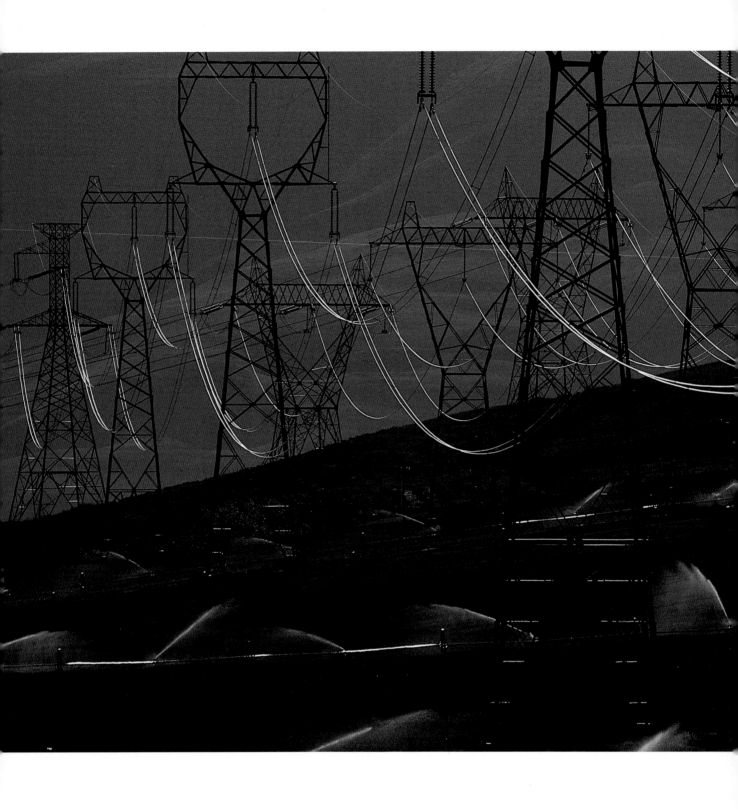

| LEARNING
TO SEE
CREATIVELY

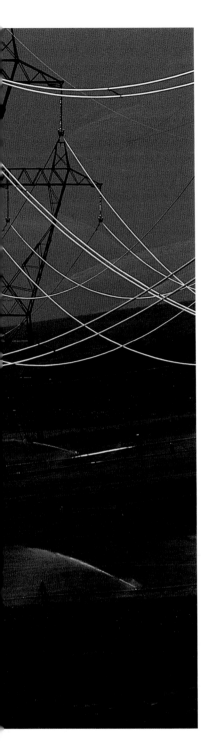

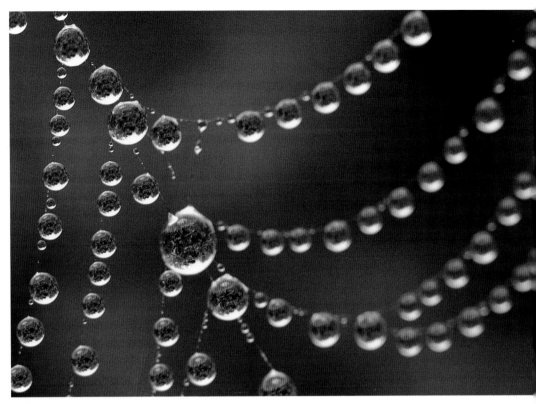

Like many photographers anxious to shoot a beautiful landscape, I have often complained about "the @#*&%#@*$@! powerlines." Ironically, in 1986 I found myself under contract to shoot "beautiful pictures of powerlines." How did I shoot successful pictures of a subject I had scorned for so long? ◆ Changing my attitude was the first step.

Second, I called upon my experiences with similar subjects, such as this spiderweb in my garden, and soon found myself applying the same visual principles to make this beautiful picture of powerlines. Curvilinear lines signify motion, growth, meandering direction, and restfulness regardless of whether they are in the natural or industrial world.

Shape

Shape is more fundamental than form, texture, or pattern because shape is the principal element of identification. You may think you smell a fragrant rose, but until you actually see its shape, you can't make a positive identification. You may hear a sexy voice on the radio, but unless you see the speaker, who knows if he or she looks sexy?

Horror movies play off our anxiety about the shape of the unseen and most have a standard script: John and Jane Doe live peacefully and quietly with their kids on Main Street until one day when a monster begins to terrorize them. Soon the police are called in, and then the fun begins. Standing in the living room with his note pad in hand, the policeman asks the family, "Can anyone describe this thing for me? Was it tall, short, fat, skinny, round, stocky, or broad?" (All of these are references to shape.) The family responds in unison. "We didn't actually see it." "But I smelled it," says one little Doe, "and it smelled like a sewer." "I heard it grunt, groan, and shriek," says Mrs. Doe. "It brushed by me in the dark hallway. I felt its slimy, coarse surface," says Mr. Doe. "And as it headed out the back door, I caught a glimpse of its bluish-purple back," says the other little Doe. Since no one saw it, the policeman is left with a description of a monster that is bluish-purple, smells like a sewer, and feels like coarse sandpaper dipped in Vaseline. The audience wants the monster captured, too, because seeing its shape would finally alleviate everyone's anxiety. Maybe that's why it is so hard to make a successful sequel to a horror movie—the audience already knows the monster's shape and is thus less easy to manipulate.

Without line there can be no shape since a shape is simply a line that is closed. Squares and rectangles are shapes enclosed by four lines, and these figures evoke feelings of stability. They symbolize the man-made world. A triangle is enclosed by three lines. In bridge and frame construction the strongest bearing members are made of three girders connected in a triangular shape. Triangular compositions echo this strength. Reminiscent of mountains and the Great Pyramids, triangles evoke feelings of permanence, endurance, weight, and dominance. But if you turn a triangle upside down onto its tip, note how the mood shifts. With the weight of the figure supported by a delicate point the triangle's message changes to instability, lightness, impermanence, and inferiority.

Curvilinear shapes, such as the letter S, evoke a sense of subtle motion, growth, and restfulness and symbolize water, plant growth, and music. The letters "SSSSSSSSSS" are much quieter and more peaceful than the louder, angular letters "VVVVVVV-VVV." When curves begin to turn back on themselves, spirals and circles appear. A circle is a line that returns to its origin by always maintaining the same distance from a central point. Of all the universal symbols in art and nature, none is stronger than the circle. It symbolizes the sun, moon, earth, and all the planets, and it evokes feelings of completion, universality, psychological wholeness, and warmth. A circle is a satisfying whole that can unify a composition by providing a center of power.

There are several things to remember when you compose a photograph that depends primarily on shapes. First, a shape is best defined when frontlit or backlit. (When the subject is frontlit, you are choosing to shoot it head on.) In addition, there should be strong contrast between the shape and its surroundings. If you want to shoot silhouettes, remember that just before and several minutes after sunrise and sunset, form and texture vanish from backlit subjects, and only stark outlines and profiles are apparent against the sky. The silhouette is the purest of all shapes, so it is not surprising that silhouettes are the most popular shapes to shoot as subject matter.

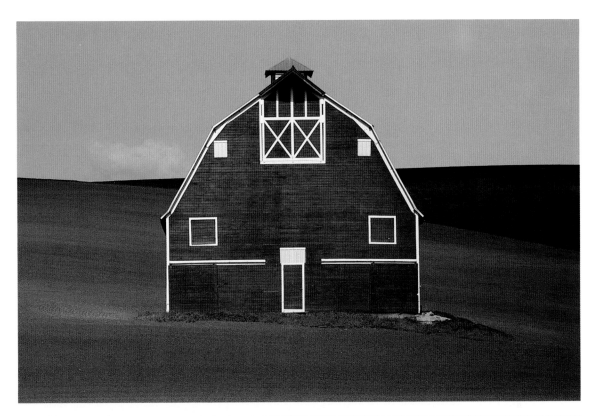

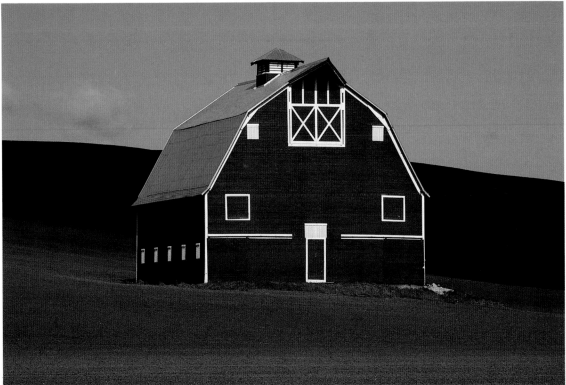

While on assignment in eastern Washington, I came upon a barn surrounded by a freshly tilled field. Wishing to record only the barn's shape, I framed only the frontlit portion and flattened the perspective even further by using my 105mm telephoto lens. As a result, I created an illusion of a single-walled barn that looks like a Hollywood movie set. If you didn't have the second picture for reference, you couldn't tell whether or not this was a real barn. ◆ Photographing shape is commonly done when the subject is backlit, but as this picture demonstrates, you can also showcase shape, provided that the shape is frontlit, you are shooting head on, and you use a telephoto lens.

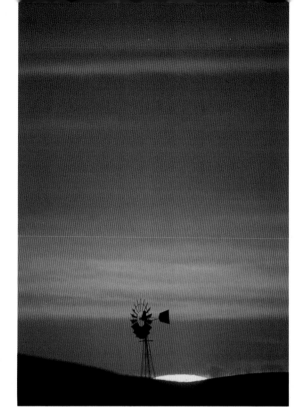

Photographers all over the world favor sunrises and sunsets as backgrounds for showcasing shapes. Whether you are in the city, country, the desert, or along the coast, there are countless shapes filling the sky above the horizon. ◆ The night before I took these pictures, I arrived in an area of eastern Oregon that was new to me. The following morning, I began scouting the horizon about forty-five minutes before sunrise by driving up and down the local country roads. At this hour of the day, it is very easy to spot interesting shapes to photograph above the horizon line as the predawn sky separates itself from the darker landscape.

◆ Soon I spotted a windmill that seemed perfectly aligned with the upcoming sunrise. To me a windmill symbolizes family and togetherness, and I thought combining this symbol with the sunrise would emphasize these qualities since the sun is also symbolic of wholeness, unity, and warmth.

◆ Ascribing to the principle that the bigger the shape, the more believable its symbolism, I chose to shoot the sunrise with a 1200mm super telephoto. Securely mounted on my tripod, the lens magnified the size of the sun and the picture's emotions as well.

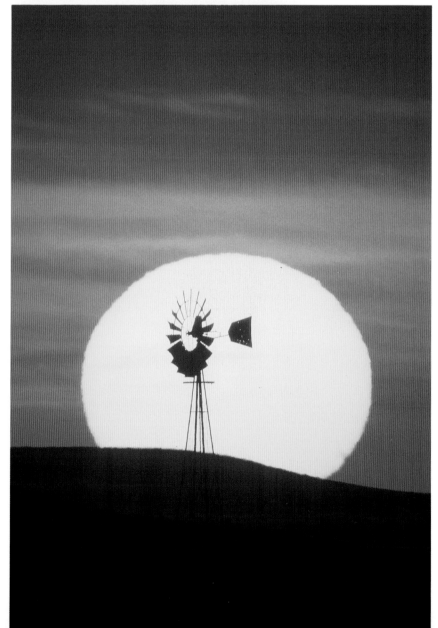

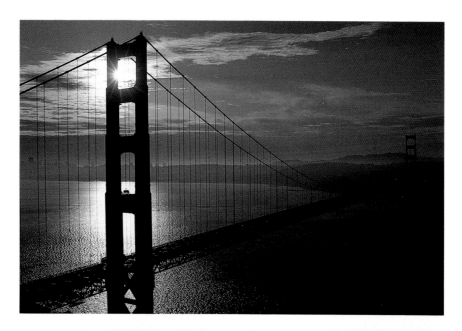

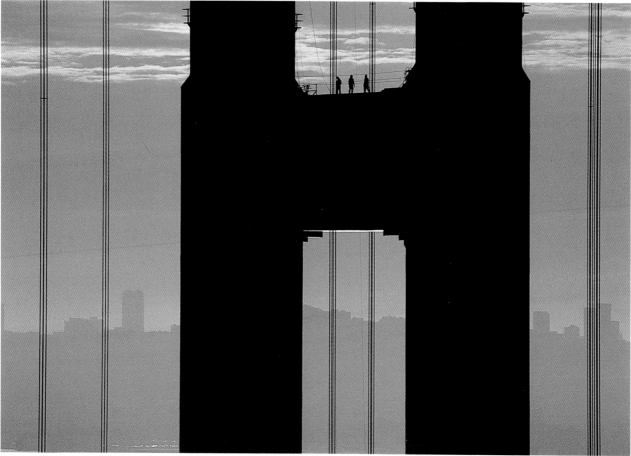

For the past three years I've been actively searching for shapes and lines that look like letters from the alphabet. I was in San Francisco shooting the Golden Gate Bridge when I discovered the letter "H." With my 300mm lens mounted on my tripod I discovered an unexpected bonus: three painters working on the H's horizontal bar. No shape is more dynamic than the human form. Nothing even comes close to resembling it. Including human shapes in this composition proved especially effective since they add a powerful sense of scale to an otherwise neutral scene. ◆ Someday I hope to publish a book of alphabet pictures. Underneath each letter will be a descriptive word or phrase that begins with the letter and conveys the mood of the picture or pertains directly to it. For example, this letter H might stand for heavy-duty, heavyweight, high-level, highfalutin, high rise, or maybe even hideout.

Form

In its purest state, a form is a shape that is sidelit. The contrast between the light and dark areas of sidelit shapes gives them form. Basically, a subject that has form is seen in three dimensions, while a shape has only two dimensions. Form assures us that an object has depth and exists in the real world. Because forms depend on light and shadow for depth, they are best photographed under sunny skies.

Squares, rectangles, triangles, and circles evoke different emotional responses. When these shapes take on form, their message is amplified. Round, curving shapes represent wholeness; yet when sidelit as forms, they often resemble parts of the human body and elicit sensual feelings. Rectangles, squares, and triangles are hard-edged shapes and when given form, they suggest the man-made world. Besides triangular mountain tops, these forms are seldom seen in nature. Hard-edged forms are interpreted as aggressive, decisive, and rigid, whereas organic forms feel quieter, lighter, and more free flowing.

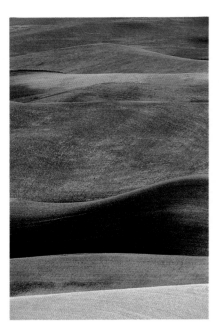 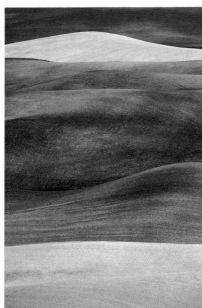 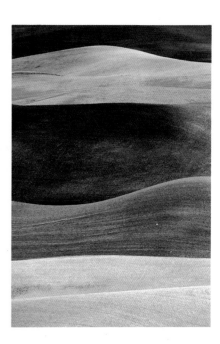

While shooting these springtime wheat fields in eastern Washington's Palouse country, I sat back for several minutes and enjoyed nature's own light show. The sky was filled with puffy clouds, lingering from the previous night's rain shower, and as each cloud passed beneath the sun, a big shadow fell across the landscape.

◆ Working with my 105mm lens from a high vantage point atop a hill, I rapidly photographed these three pictures of the same rolling hills. Every press of the shutter revealed a new and different composition as the passing clouds dragged dark shadows in and out of the scene, creating new images for the camera to record.

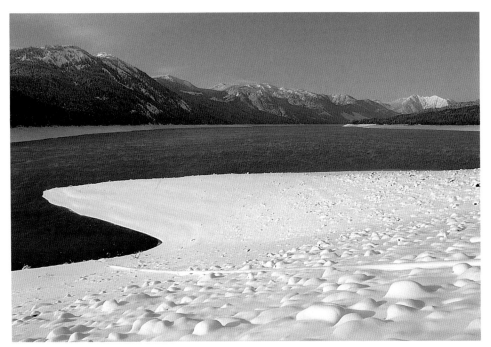

I was on an assignment shooting dams and reservoirs for the Army Corps of Engineers when one reservoir near the Idaho-Washington border caught my attention. The rocks dotting the reservoir's edge had been transformed by the wind and snow into marvelous, curving shapes that, viewed through my 200mm lens, reminded me of the human form. Finding the right combination of forms to express my intention wasn't easy, but this picture says it all—sensuality.

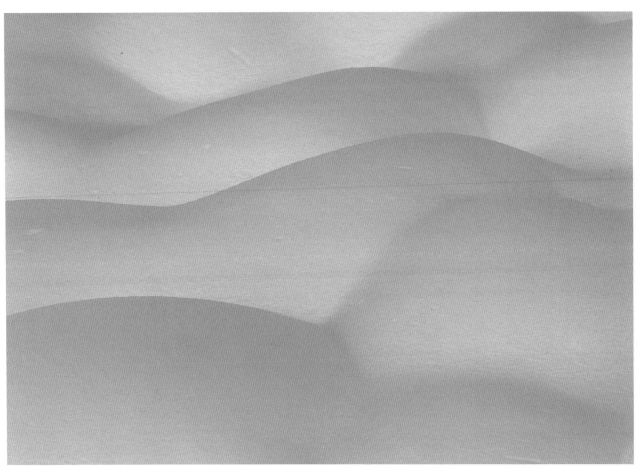

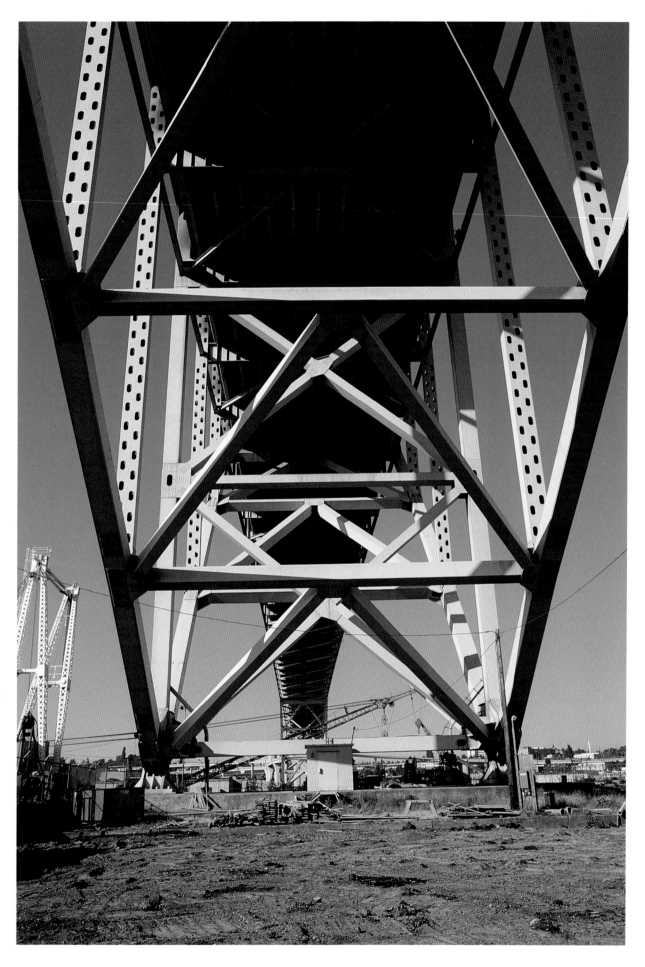

I am especially fond of bridges, as long as they are not the old-fashioned covered type. I experience bridges as being strong and forceful; paradoxically, many parts of a bridge are light and delicate. Perhaps the tension this sets up explains my love for them. ◆ Portland, Oregon's Fremont Bridge, shown on the left, is among my favorites. I used my 400mm lens to pull out a small section of its form from its supporting girders. Compare this top picture with the closeup of the feather. Although the girder and the feather fill the same amount of space inside the frame and were both composed on the diagonal, the picture of the girder has more visual weight. The girder itself doesn't create this feeling, nor does the feather lack anything essential for composing a strong image. The difference comes from the contrast between a natural and a man-made subject—we respond to artificial shapes differently than we do to organic ones.

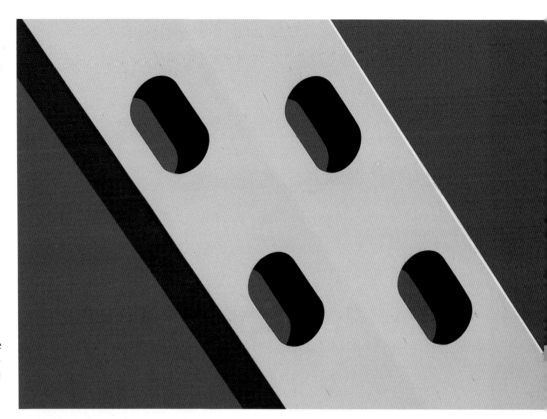

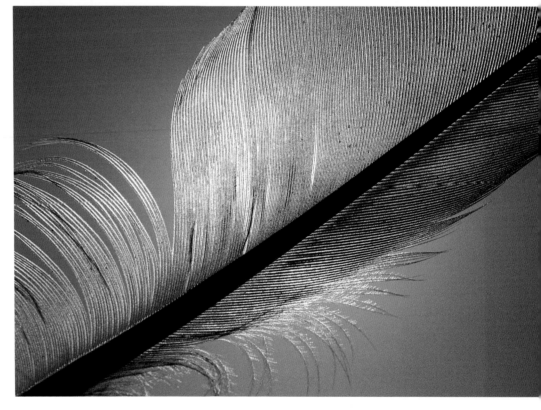

Texture

Even if you've never been thrown from a bicycle, the thought of skidding hands and face down across the pavement can still send chills down your spine. Evoking texture, or the way a surface feels, is a powerful stimulus for arousing old memories; so when texture dominates a composition, the picture invites a high degree of viewer response. As newborn babies, most of us discovered texture long before any other sensation. During our first years, we probably scurried and scooted across floors made of hardwood, concrete, tile, carpet, dirt, and gravel; and when mom wasn't looking (or chose not to panic), we may have sampled handfuls of mud, grass, paper, fabric, sawdust, and dry dog food. Some of these experiences with texture were pleasant; others were not. We learned to prefer soft, smooth, and silky things and steer clear of rough, coarse, and jagged surfaces. As we grew older, these perceptions about texture were reinforced by a slew of positive and negative adjectives found in our daily language. For example, a woman's "soft" voice may arouse delicate feelings, but a man's "gravelly" voice may elicit aggression. A "hard"-nosed manager seldom wins the affection of his workers, whereas the "smooth"-talking manager usually does. "Sharply" dressed people "cut" good figures; "dull" appearances and "dull" movies don't "impress" us and "barely make a dent" in our consciousness.

There are many ways to use texture effectively. For example, you could lie down on a sandy beach or pebbled lakeshore and with your wide-angle lens fill the foreground with looming pebbles; the resulting pictures would immediately arouse the viewer's sense of touch. If you fill a picture frame with broken glass, jagged rocks, or soap bubbles from the kitchen sink, you'll reawaken the viewer's own experiences with these textures. The way you light a subject plays a major role in conveying its texture. Sidelighting is definitely the best technique to use for highlighting textured surfaces for the camera.

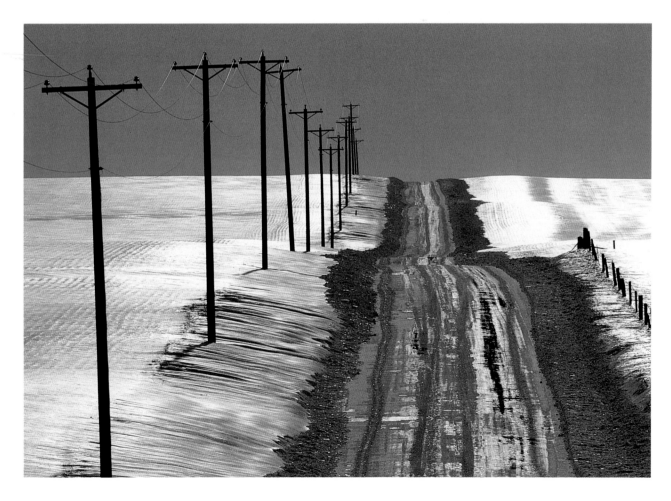

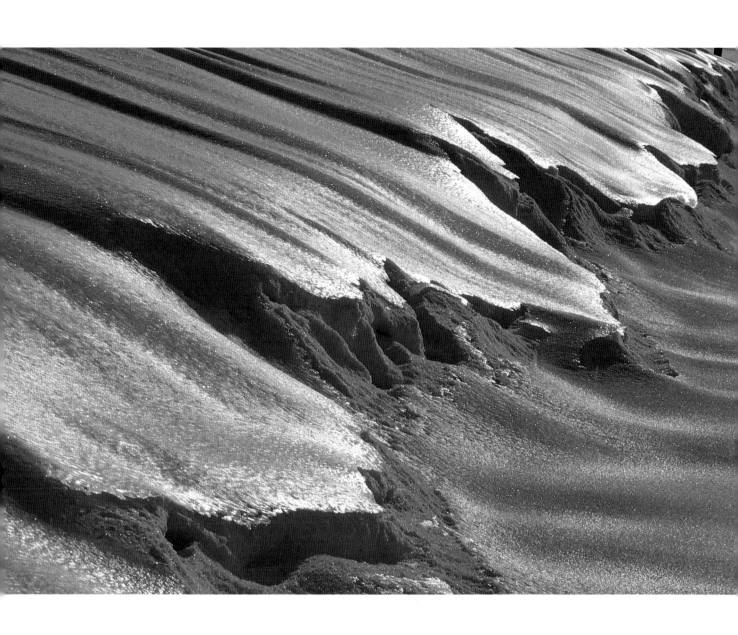

I love shooting in eastern Oregon during the winter months. The combination of snow, ice, and cloudy days sets up a monochromatic condition that speaks volumes about loneliness and solitude. This empty road seemed to sum up the mood I was after—cold, stark, and lonely. But before moving on, I composed some closeups of the road's edge with my 200mm lens because I was intrigued by its texture and the feelings of caution it elicited. Imagine walking on this slippery, jagged surface— each step would have to be carefully planned to avoid slipping and falling on the hard ice.

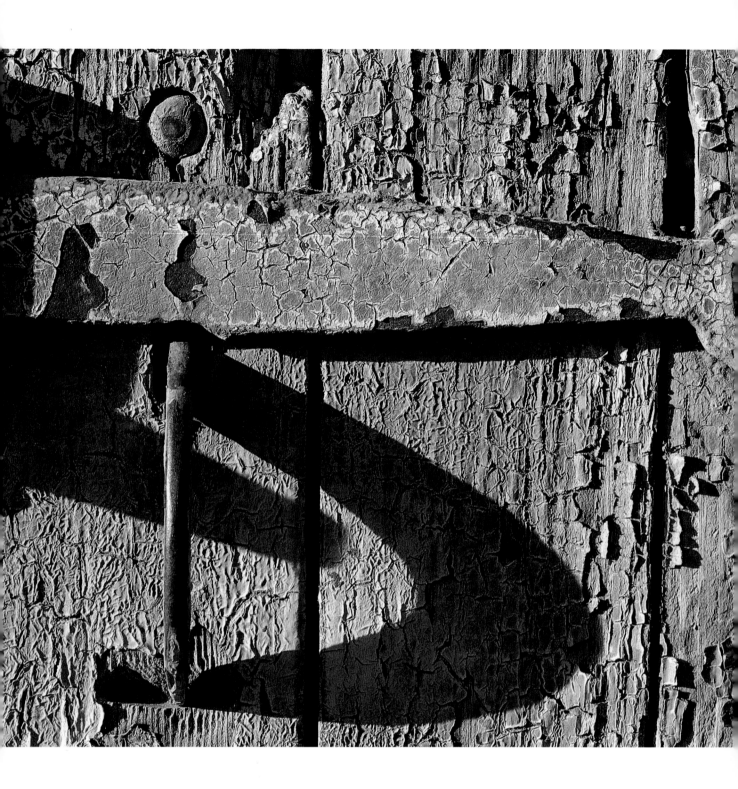

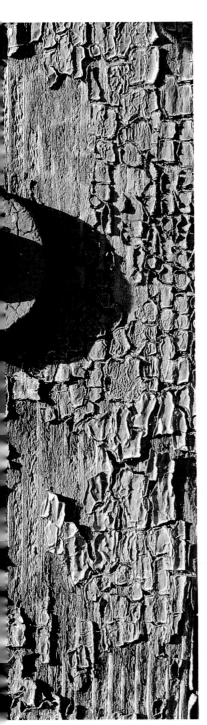

After an early morning shoot in eastern Washington, I came upon this old garage. It was alive with texture, so I set up my camera on a tripod, and with my 35–70mm lens in its macro setting, I zeroed in on this old door latch.

◆ The texture you see in the closeup on the left was totally dependent on sidelighting. The other closeup picture, which I took the following morning under an overcast sky, is flat and lifeless in comparison.

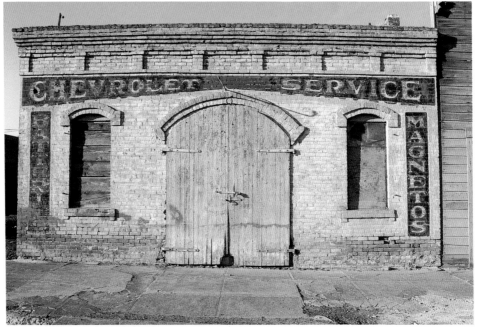

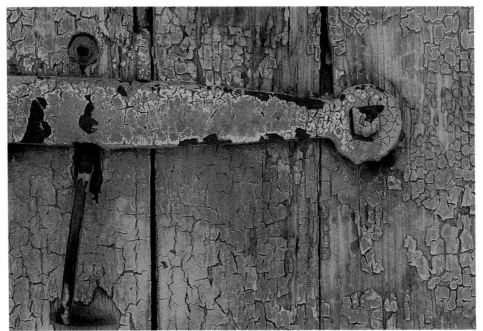

While waiting for sunset on an Oregon beach, I ventured toward a group of rocks bathed by water falling from a drain pipe. I became so fascinated with their smooth texture that I forgot all about shooting the sunset behind me; instead, I shot the rocks with my 105mm lens and a tripod. ◆ This closeup illustrates how our response to texture is entirely based on emotion. Because these rocks are smooth, most of us will have positive feelings about them. But if we think about it, smooth rocks are just as hard and potentially hazardous as jagged ones.

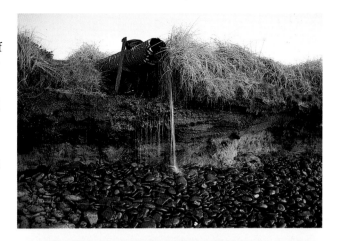

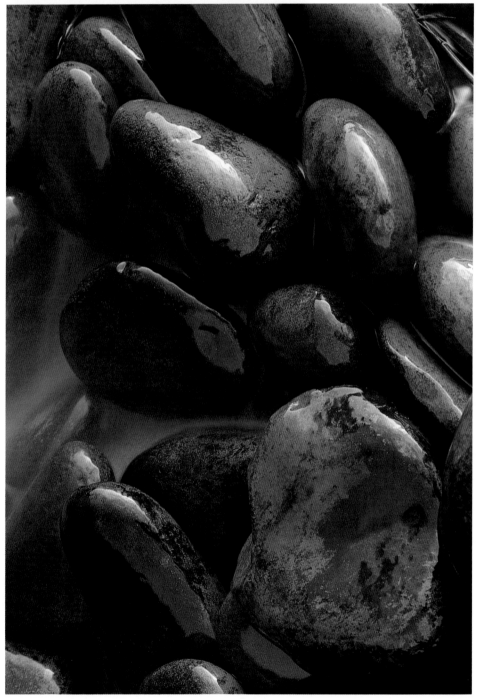

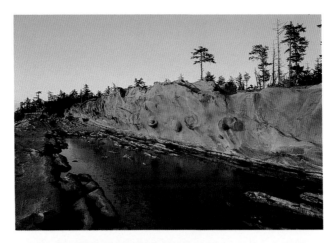

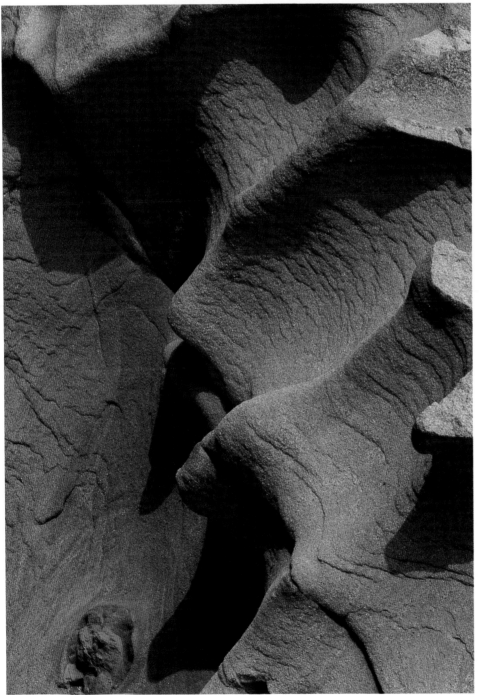

During another outing along the Oregon coast, I found my hopes for shooting a sunset disappearing as the sun headed for a large bank of fog on the horizon; but as the saying goes, "When life gives you lemons, make lemonade." Instead of loading up my gear and calling it a day, I decided to search for texture in this sandstone wall. ◆ Looking up and down the sandstone wall with my 200mm telephoto mounted on a tripod, the lens led me to this composition. The low-angled sidelighting from the late afternoon sun warmed the wall's undulating surface, making it more touchable. No matter how the picture is turned, its sensual appeal creates the same emotional response. Ahhh!—the joy of shooting texture.

Pattern

When lines, shapes, forms, or textures are repeated over and over in more or less regular intervals, a pattern is created. Looking down from a rooftop, you can see that the cars filling a parking lot make a pattern. Walking through a grocery store's aisles usually reveals patterns of canned goods stacked on the shelves. Whatever emotional response a single design element arouses is multiplied when it is repeated in a pattern. Patterns amplify the symbolism of their components, turning up a picture's volume, so to speak. People are generally fascinated by such repetition, and many of the arts—poetry and music, for instance—rely heavily upon it. No wonder that we are also attracted to visual patterns; the order they present us with is oddly comforting, even when their message is abrasive.

Paying attention to any composition is critical, but if developing a pattern is your sole intent, you must fill your entire frame with it. Using a macro or telephoto lens can help introduce order in your composition since either lens will reduce your depth of field and thereby narrow your perspective. If you use a wide-angle lens, you must choose a point of view that keeps the camera's film plane parallel to the subject; otherwise, the units of pattern in the foreground will be larger than those in the background, resulting in a visual effect that gradually recedes from the viewer and therefore diminishes in emotional impact.

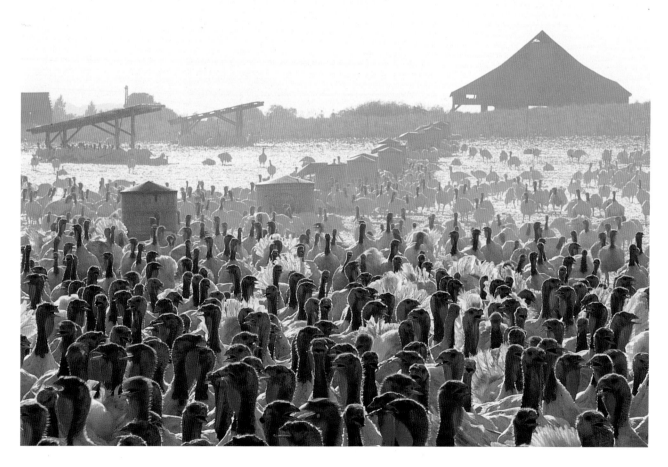

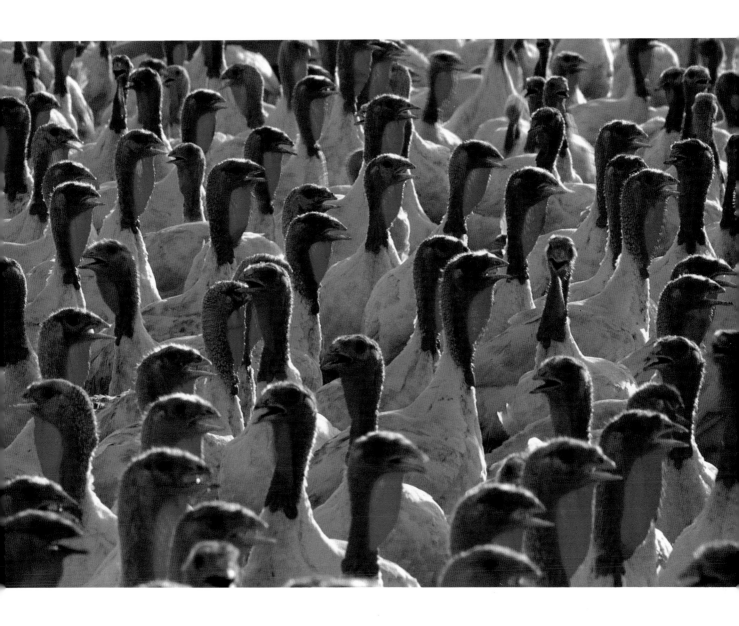

A farmer who lives a few miles from my home raises turkeys. I've driven by his farm many times, but only once have I seen the sun backlighting the birds. That was the day I took these pictures. Screeching my car to a halt, I wasted very little time setting up—I mounted my 300mm lens on a tripod and started ex- posing one humorous pic- ture of pattern after another. ◆ When I switched to a 35mm me- dium–wide-angle lens, I lessened the overall impact of the turkey's pattern in the composition on the left. Note how the birds in the foreground are more vibrant than those in the distance, an effect caused by the wide-angle lens.

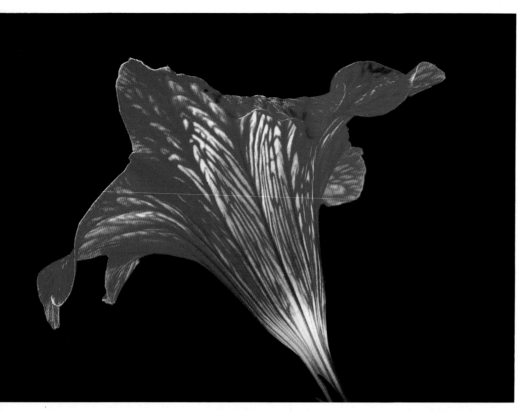

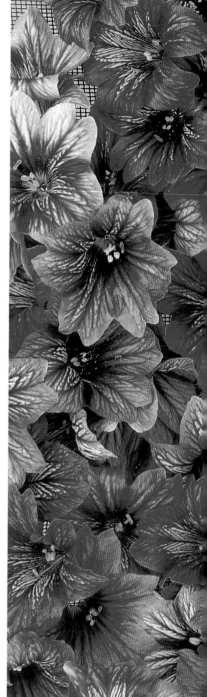

A shaft of light from a low-angled sun traveled through the open door of my greenhouse and backlit this flower much the same way a spotlight pinpoints a soloist onstage. The glowing flower caught my attention, and I decided to heighten the sun's effect by photographing my subject from a point of view that would place it in front of a background of open shade. ◆ There was a four-stop difference between the open shade and the flower. Using a 55mm macro lens, I adjusted my exposure for the brightly lit flower, thus ensuring that the background would go black. The strong contrast in the composition certainly called attention to the single flower; however, I decided to amplify the flower's impact by filling an entire picture frame from edge to edge with a pattern based on this type of flower. ◆ The following morning, I went into the garden and picked a big bunch of the same species. Inside the greenhouse I pulled the blossoms off the stems and set the flowers upright on a wire screen. The diffused light filtering through the fiberglass walls illuminated my subjects in a soft, even light. Once everything was arranged, I climbed up a small stepladder and shot straight down at the flowers with my 50mm normal lens.

◆ More than any photograph I've taken, this pattern picture leaves viewers divided between those who don't like it at all because the pattern of the brightly colored flowers is too jarring and those who think the pattern is simply wonderful. What do you think?

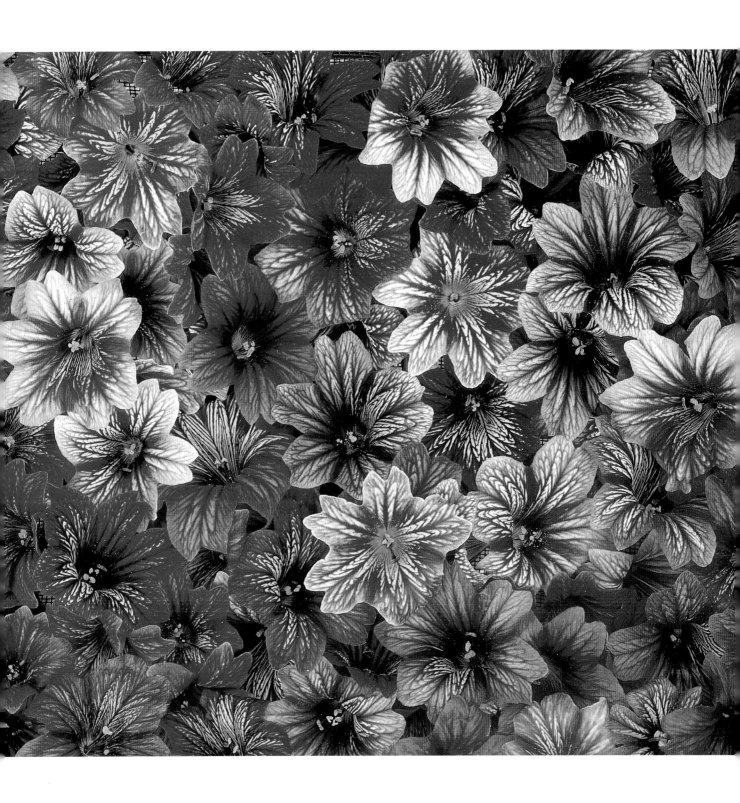

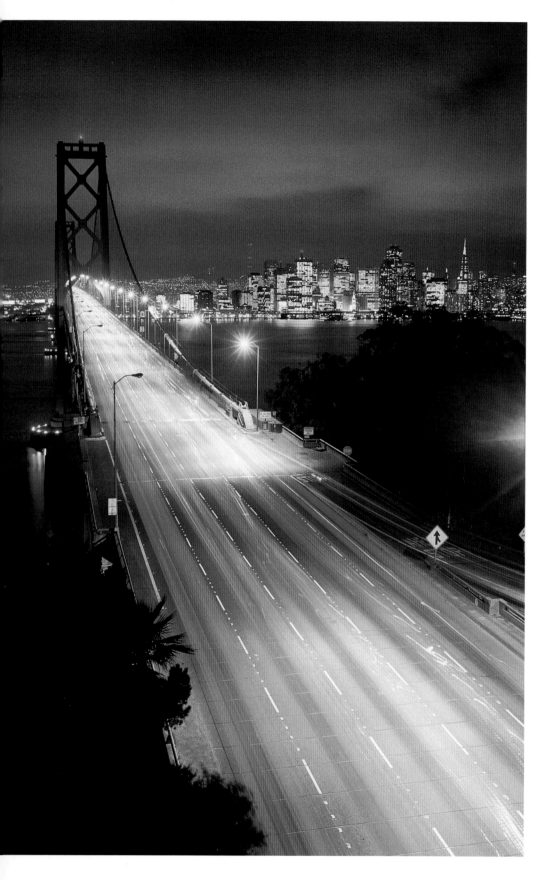

Treasure Island is one of the most popular places for shooting pictures of San Francisco. Putting the Bay Bridge in the foreground and the city's skyline off to the right, as I have done here, is a typical picture composition. On the evening I took these pictures I was on the prowl for abstract images. I climbed a hill directly above the tunnel of traffic going to and from the island in order to isolate the lanes of traffic with my 400mm lens.

◆ The resulting photograph demonstrates the arresting power of pattern. The lines of moving traffic subtly converge at the top of the frame, which makes the viewer feel the flow of traffic is from the bottom of the frame toward the top. But if you turn the photograph upside down, the feeling changes. Now the traffic appears to be coming down at you. This illusion of movement can be applied to other subjects as well.

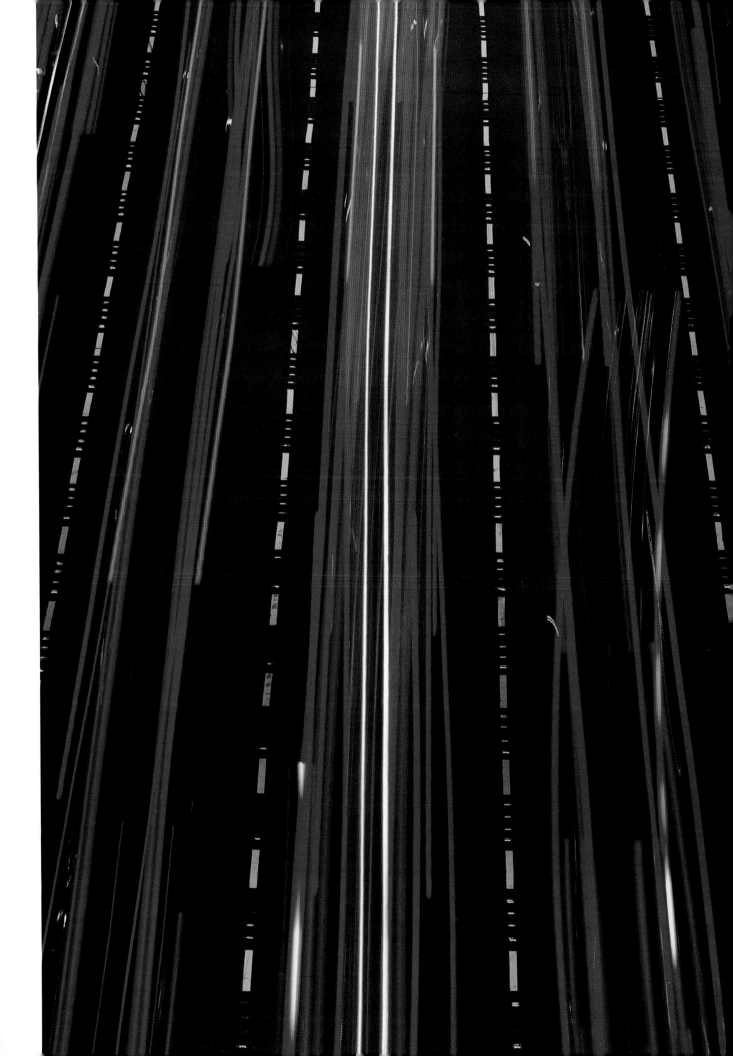

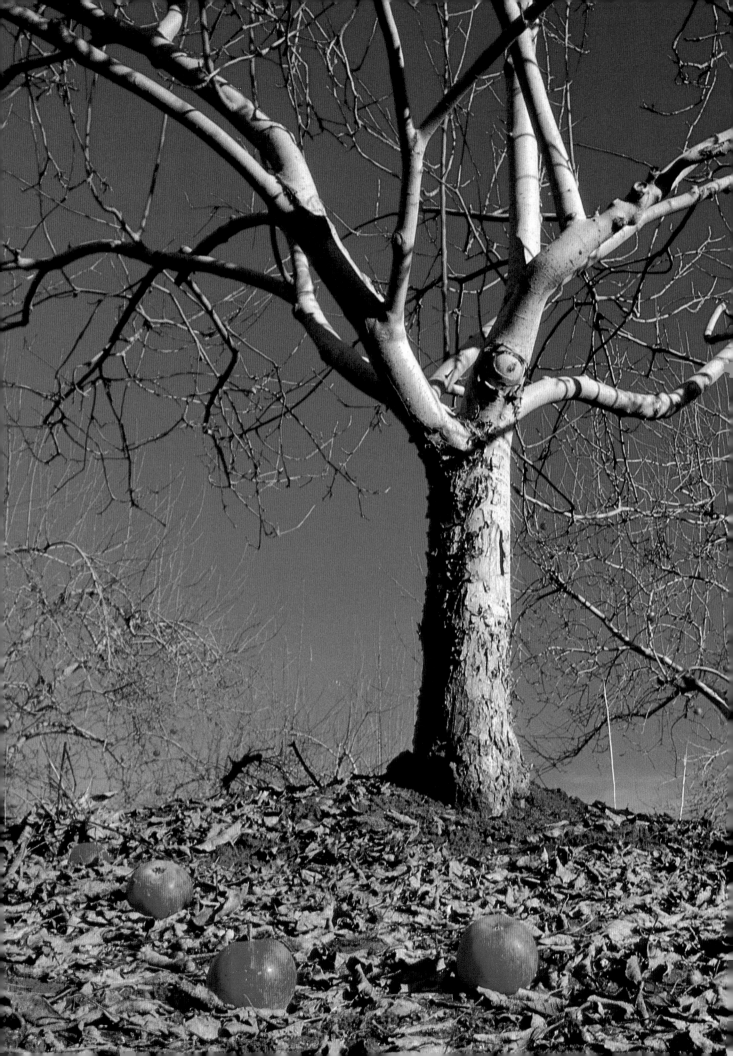

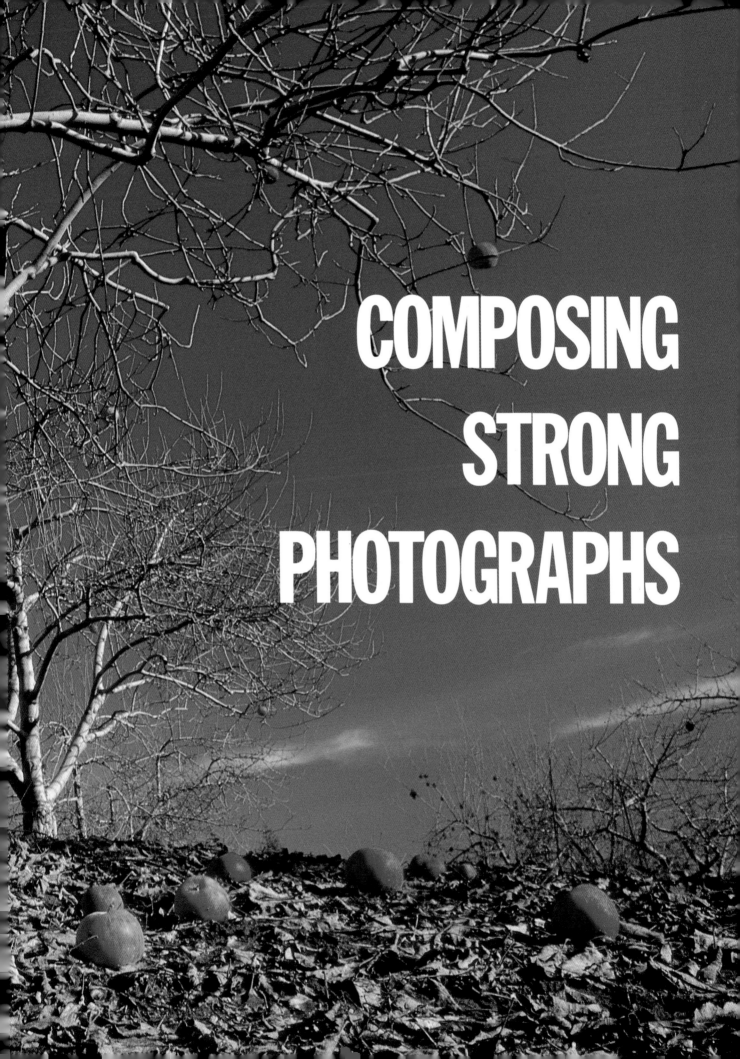

COMPOSING STRONG PHOTOGRAPHS

The marvelous partnership between the eye and the brain is mutually stimulating and seems to keep both always on the move. Whenever you stare at a fixed spot, your eyes jerk around the area surrounding it, creating a changing pattern on the retina for your brain to interpret. Viewing an entire picture, the eyes flicker wildly as they pick out the most interesting areas. Why does one picture hold your attention for a long time, while another only musters a fleeting glance? Some photographers say making a compelling picture is a matter of using the right f-stop, the right exposure, or the right lens, and frequently you'll hear that success depends on finding the right subject. All of these strategies are important in successful image making; however, the only way to make a good picture is to design the right composition. Without it, a picture's impact will be diminished or lost, no matter how provocative the subject is.

Both visually and mentally, human beings demand order. This is basic to the laws of nature and underscores the Gestalt theory of visual perception. In your daily life you organize your time, your priorities, and your checking account, and when they are not orderly, you feel stressed. Good books, good music, and good pictures also rely on internal order, and they include only enough material to convey the artist's subject, theme, or intent.

The two major principles of composition are simplicity and tension. Simplifying a picture's visual elements helps to satisfy the viewer's need to identify the subject. Simplicity is easily achieved when you organize your subject inside the frame in a clear and concise manner. Tension arises from the interplay between a picture's visual elements, and this produces its tone and makes it interesting. For example, a picture can have a gentle, a decisive, or a forceful tone, depending on how its elements are organized, or balanced against each other.

What are some of the ways to achieve greater simplicity in your pictures? The most common solution is to walk closer to your subject. Often a picture fails because its subject is too small in the frame. By way of analogy, when you stand at the back of a crowded union hall, you can't hear the speaker's voice. Likewise, you shut the viewer out of a picture when the subject isn't close enough. Walk closer to it, and watch how the four sides of the viewing frame delete the extraneous material overpowering it.

Changing lenses is another way to bring order to a composition. Because a telephoto lens has a narrow angle of view, it is the best lens for cutting through clutter, and its ability to bring objects closer increases a subject's importance. In addition, the telephoto can transform a distracting background into a monocolor backdrop via the len's shallow depth of

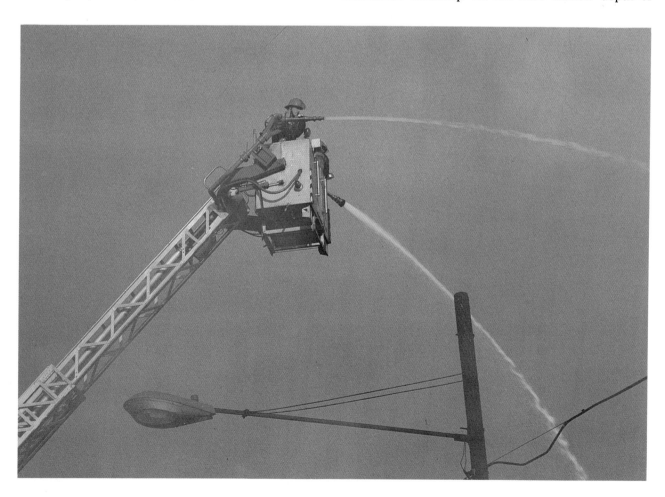

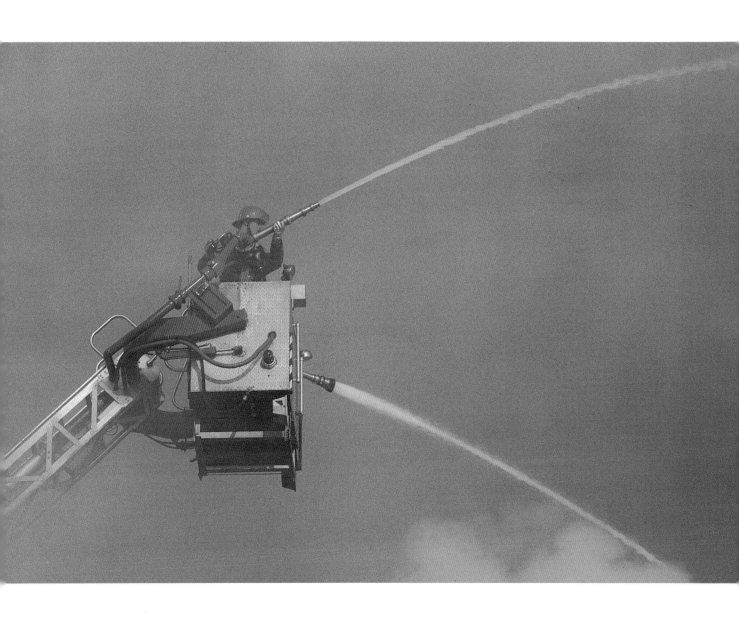

I had just started my car and turned on the radio when I heard the news about a five-alarm fire underway on the other side of town. My plans were to head into Portland and shoot the sunrise, but since I had never shot a fire before, I decided to check it out. Within a few minutes of my arrival, I was shooting away rapidly with my 80–200mm zoom and was intently focused on the lefthand image of a fireman in his bucket. Several exposures later, I realized that the street light was in the way. ◆ By moving a few feet to the left and zooming into a longer telephoto range, I was able to crop out the pole, thereby improving the composition. Because our eyes tend to follow movement from left to right, I chose to place the fireman on the left. The action of the water hoses leads the eye throughout the rest of the frame. ◆ Like many other compositions in this book, the top one works not because of what is shown, but because of what the picture suggests. You don't need to see bright orange flames or a burning structure to figure out that this fireman is fighting a fire.

field at wide-open apertures. On the other hand, a wide-angle lens is useful for showing more of a scene. Although it is seldom used for single-subject compositions, using a wide-angle lens is ideal when the composition has a panoramic story to tell.

Changing your point of view can also enhance a composition's simplicity. Getting down low in relation to your subject increases the size and importance of any foreground matter. In addition, by simply changing your point of view, you may be able to hide unwanted material or merge it against the background.

Employing selective focus means choosing a point of view that allows you to focus through the immediate foreground. This technique, which involves using a large lens opening, throws the foreground out of focus, thereby placing greater emphasis on your subject. Selective focus works best in high-contrast situations, so look for light and dark areas, sunlight and shadows. Choose a background that is darker than your subject and expose for the subject exclusively; the resulting background will throw the emphasis onto your subject.

Our world is fast paced and constantly changing. Day by day, we respond positively to certain stimuli;

meanwhile, we subconsiously block out useless input. But the camera cannot abstract information. Regardless of the subject chosen, the camera records everything around it inside the picture frame. That is why so many pictures taken by amateurs are unattractive and chaotic. Since no one likes to look at messy compositions, these pictures end up in the wastebasket instead of in the winner's circle.

To improve your pictures you need to become acutely aware of how you organize your subject matter; only then can the camera effectively record your intentions. You may find it helpful to approach new compositions by quietly reminding yourself, "Before I press the shutter, I will inspect all four corners of the frame and be certain that only pertinent subject matter is included." Nine times out of ten, you'll make the conscious discovery that you need to move closer or farther back, or that you need to get down low, move up high, shift right or left, or change lenses. These are all choices that only you, the photographer, can make. Real seeing is not a function of the camera—the camera is merely a tool for viewing your subjects. How you consciously arrange them on the film is a creative act left up to you.

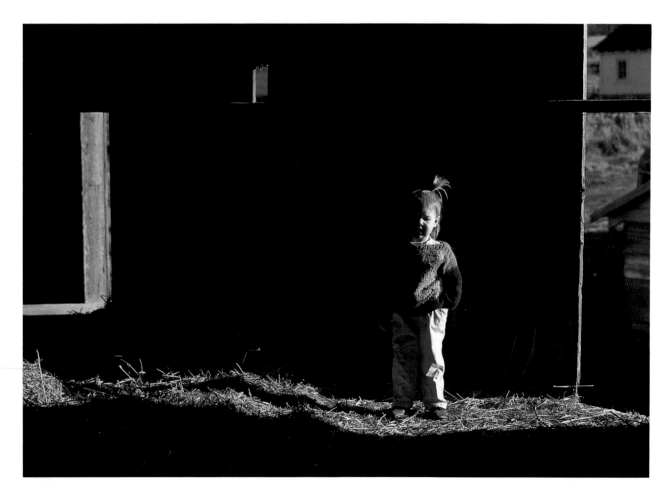

One sunny morning, my niece and I walked up the wooden ladder that leads to the hayloft in my barn. The early morning light was casting long shadows along the hayloft's floor. Using my 50–300mm zoom, I shot the picture on the left at the 50mm focal length. Although my niece is the subject, notice how the tonal contrast in this picture causes the eye to jerk around, bouncing from one highlight to the next. Such a response is similar to being in a darkened movie theatre when someone opens the exit door to the side of the stage. Your eye immediately jerks off the screen and dashes over to the light streaming in from outdoors. Unless something outdoors rivets your attention, you would probably resent the light's intrusion, just as you do in this picture. ◆ The brain's ability to compensate for extreme contrasts between light and dark make this type of compositional problem difficult to spot. Unlike the camera, the brain can see a wide range of light and dark simultaneously. Using your brain's vision, you can see into shadows quite clearly; up in the hayloft I could see the hay on the floor, the old weathered wood, and the rusty nails hanging from the wall. However, the camera doesn't have that same latitude; its vision is limited to a range of plus or minus two stops. If you were to take a light reading of this scene, you would discover a five-stop difference between the shadow and sunlit areas. Since my exposure was based on my sunlit niece, the shadows were naturally quite underexposed. ◆ Actually, such scenes are not major compositional problems; in

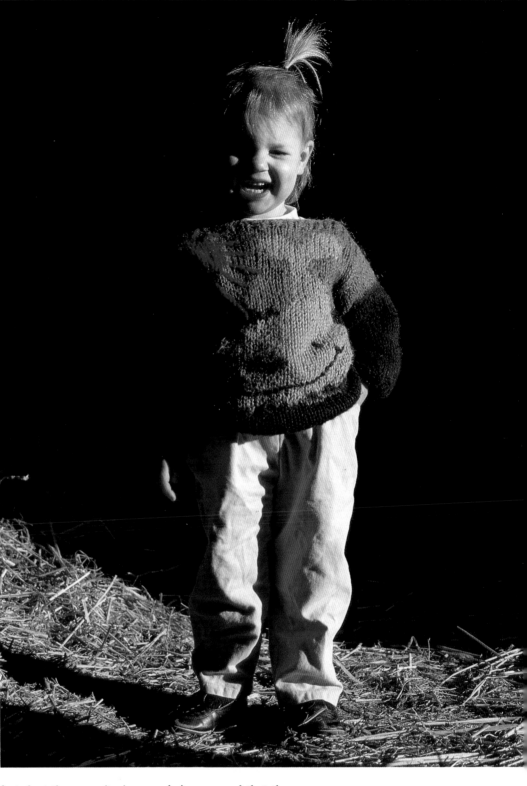

fact, just the opposite is true. You can always use light and shadow to call attention to your subject by way of tonal contrast. After zooming out to 200mm, I was able to fill the frame with my niece; in addition, my exposure choice ensured that the open shade behind her would record as a deep dark background. This difference in tonal contrast leaves no doubt in the viewer's mind that my niece is the subject not the hayloft.

Filling the Picture Frame

There are many ways to improve a composition. One is to fill the frame with your subject, thereby giving it more weight. Whether you choose to walk closer (which is by far the cheapest route) or to switch to a telephoto lens, your subject should dominate the picture area. This leaves no doubt in the viewer's mind about your intentions.

If you go through your photo album or slide file, chances are you'd discover lots of pictures that don't live up to the expectations you had for them when you pressed the shutter, generally because you weren't close enough to your subjects. It may be obvious what your intentions were, but when a subject is so small that it gets lost in the composition, the resulting pictures don't necessarily convey your intent to the viewer. Many photographers excuse these bad pictures by calling them "snapshots." But why make excuses when you know your real purpose was to capture something essential about these subjects and convey your feelings to the viewer?

Telephoto lenses are particularly good for photographing people, especially children, partly because these lenses bring subjects closer to the film without disrupting the subjects' psychological boundaries. In addition, the telephoto's flattened perspective is the most flattering for facial details, which is why the telephoto is sometimes referred to as a portrait lens.

Cluttered compositions can be a problem when shooting landscapes, too. Most landscapes are made with normal or wide-angle lenses. These lenses offer a greater angle of view, as opposed to the telephoto, and thus allow more clutter to enter the picture field. So when you shoot with wider lenses, you need to be fully conscious of everything going on inside your viewfinder. My advice for shooting landscapes is to *slow down*! Unlike doing candids of kids or action photography, shooting landscapes should be pleasureable and relaxing and seldom requires split-second thinking. Why hurry yourself when that only results in ho-hum, so-so compositions?

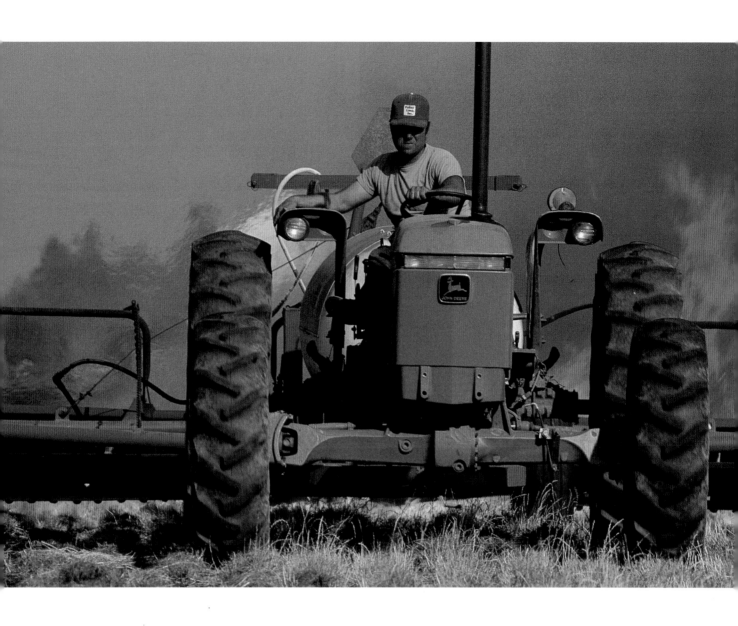

I had my camera with me when I came upon this farmer burning his field. After mounting my 400mm lens and camera on a tripod, I waited patiently for his fire-breathing machine to move closer to me and fill the frame. Then I quickly fired off several shots of the tractor. Its size and the roaring heat from the fire create tremendous impact in the composition. In addition, the compression of picture elements caused by my telephoto lens adds bulk to the already brimming frame.

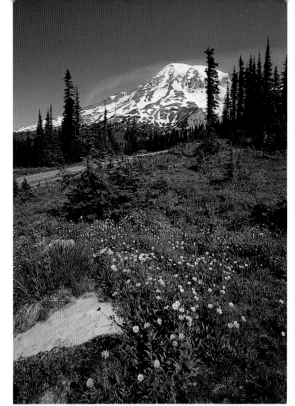

Looking at the top picture of the mountain landscape, is my photographic intent clear? You see an alpine meadow, but note the additional clutter. The nearby road, complete with the family Surburban wagon, really has no place in this composition. Including the road and car doesn't work because they symbolize the man-made world, which causes a clash in the photograph between man and nature. Since my intention was to do a composition limited to a nature theme, the road and wagon are distracting.

◆ Understand that most landscape compositions work much the same way a good book does; both have a beginning, a middle, and end expressed so that each section leads you into the next without disruption. Using this analogy, you can see that the additional story line introduced by the white-faced rock, the road, and the wagon have no bearing on the picture's theme. ◆ Removing the unnecessary elements was easy. First, I changed my position from eye level to the flower's level, which brought me down low to the ground. This made the flowers soar in the foreground, blocking out the distant road. Moving to the right allowed me to eliminate the white-faced rock. And finally, with my aperture set at $f/22$ and the focus preset via the depth-of-field scale, I was able to record sharpness throughout my entire composition. The resulting story line reads as follows, "Once upon a time, there were some beautiful, pink, mountain asters that dotted the forested meadows near the base of a tall, snow-capped peak . . . ."

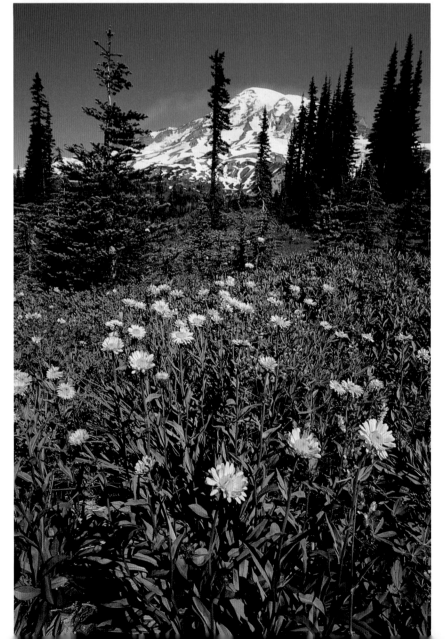

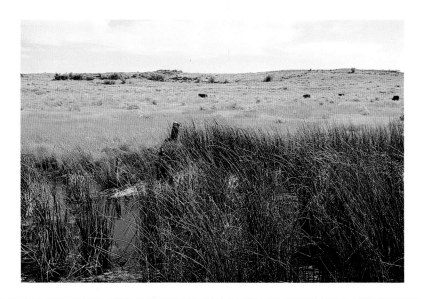

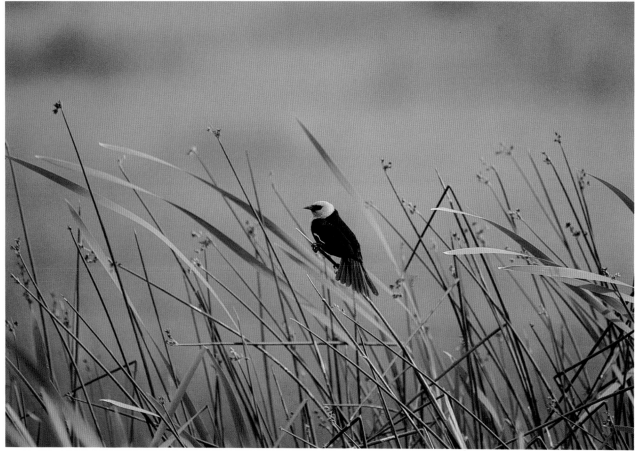

Tonal and color contrasts can be used to eliminate clutter, too. All of us have, at one time or another, photographed the proverbial "animal dot in the landscape." You swear the animal is there somewhere on your film, "Because, after all, I framed it in the camera!" I know that the top picture shows a yellow-headed blackbird in a marsh; yet you ask, "Where is it?" Due to my lens choice and the scene's lack of tonal contrast, the bird got lost. ◆ This is a classic case of the mind creating an illusion of a filled frame. As I focused on this bird with a 50mm lens, my mind enlarged the subject and told my eyes that the frame was filled. This type of mental trickery goes on all the time. You won't fall prey to such illusions if you divorce yourself from your mind's eye and instead focus solely on what is really going on in your viewfinder. ◆ With the aid of my 400mm lens I was able to bring the bird closer. And because of the telephoto's shallow depth of field, the background records as an out-of-focus green, providing the tonal contrast needed to separate it from the bird. Note that the frame is *not* filled with the bird but rather with opposing contrasts. This focuses your interest on the bird.

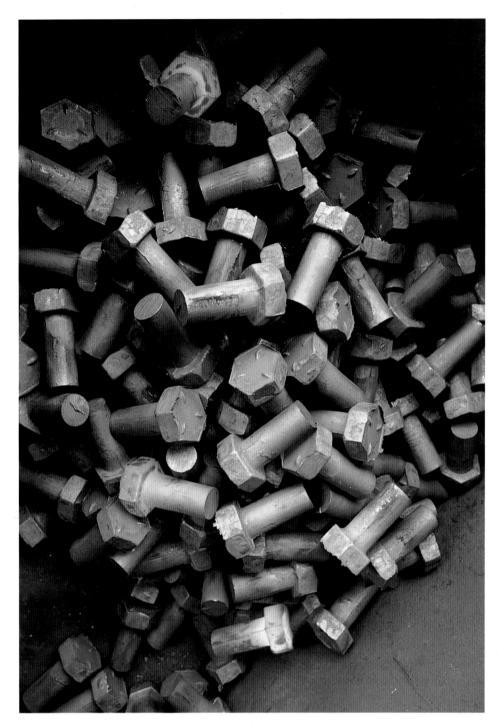

On assignment for a foundry, I was looking for one composition to sum up the company's operations. After several hours of shooting, I came upon a metal container filled with large bolts hot off the press. I decided that doing a pattern shot was not feasible since the combination of the cool, gray bolts and the hot, pink bolts caused the eye to jerk around too much without discerning my intent. ◆ After several minutes of planning, I sought the help of the worker who was pressing these bolts. I borrowed a pair of large metal tongs and began to move the cooler bolts into a small area inside the bin. Using my 105mm lens and a small extension tube, I was able to fill the frame with only cool, gray bolts. I chose the 105mm and extension tube instead of my 50mm lens because the heat emanating from the bolts was too intense for me to view them up close. ◆ Once I had arranged the cooler bolts to suit my purposes inside the camera's viewfinder, I asked the worker to place a red-hot bolt carefully on a diagonal across the gray bolts. This separation by color clearly calls attention to the red-hot bolt, and its diagonal positioning creates a feeling of movement in the composition.

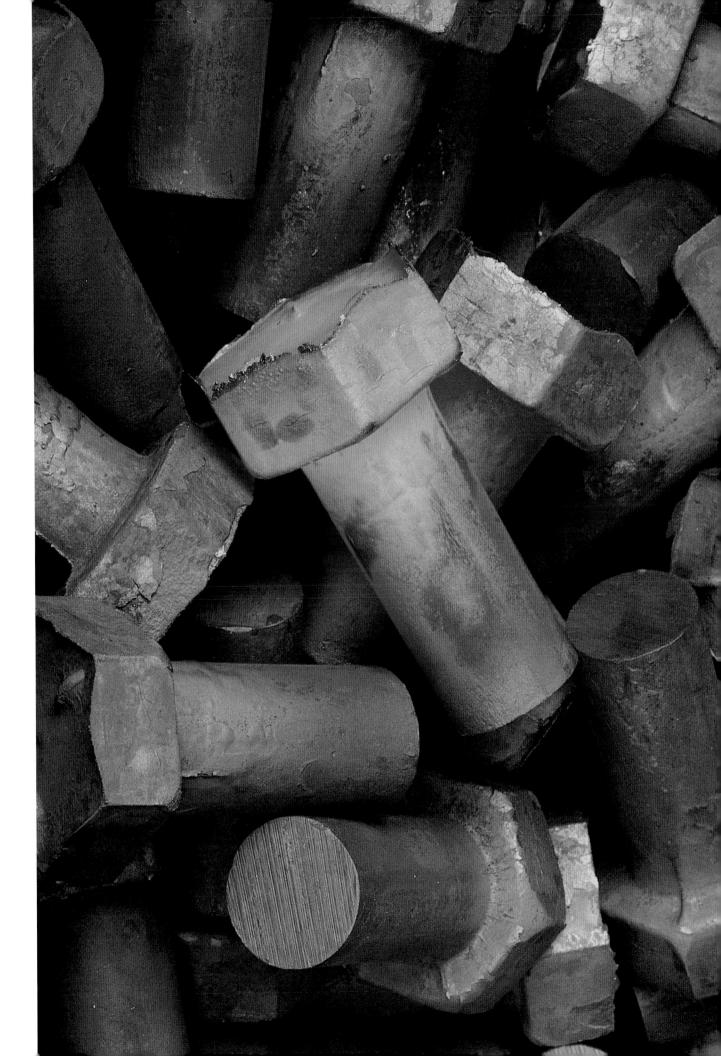

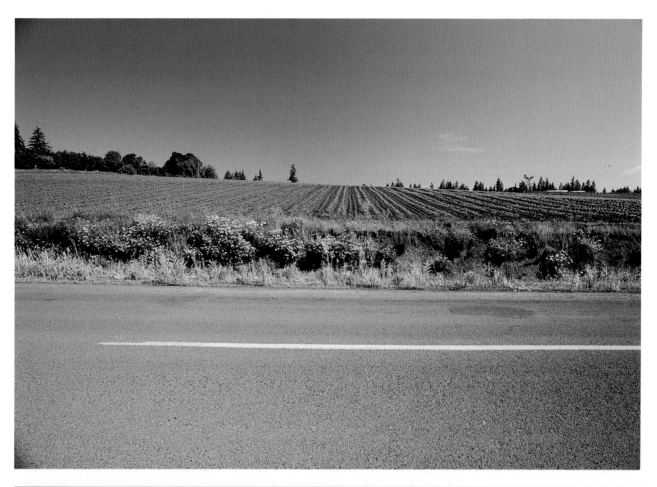

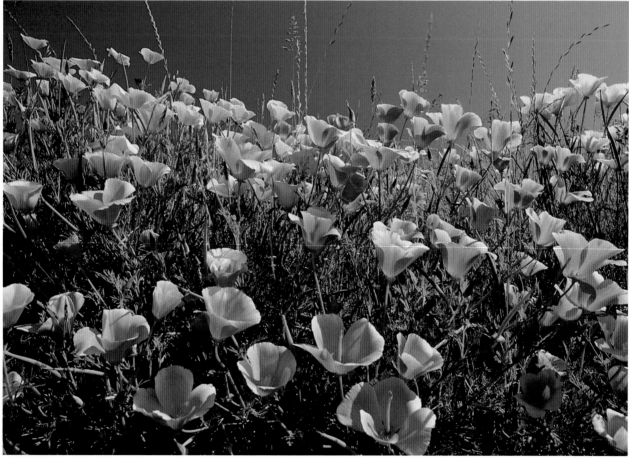

| LEARNING
TO SEE
CREATIVELY

From across the road where I'd just finished a midmorning snack and a cup of coffee, I spotted this roadside ditch of California poppies. I decided it was a good place to practice changing lenses, shifting my point of view, and looking for tonal or color contrasts. First, using my wide-angle lens and a low viewpoint, I moved in very close and filled the frame with flowers. The unique perspective created by the wide angle gives the viewer the impression that I was shooting in a meadow brimming with thousands of poppies.

◆ Next, I switched to my 200mm lens, and with the aperture set wide open I leaned against the side of the ditch and began focusing six to eight feet into the scene, ever mindful of the other flowers and grasses in front of the lens. This selective-focus technique allowed me to separate just a few of the blooms from the crowded hillside. Notice how this effect also created tonal and color contrast in the picture. ◆ Finally, with my 55mm macro lens I spied a single bloom. I chose to showcase the flower against a shadowed background that I created by hanging my jacket from my tripod. The flower's stark yellow-orange color is even more vivid and arresting with the addition of the dark-toned background.

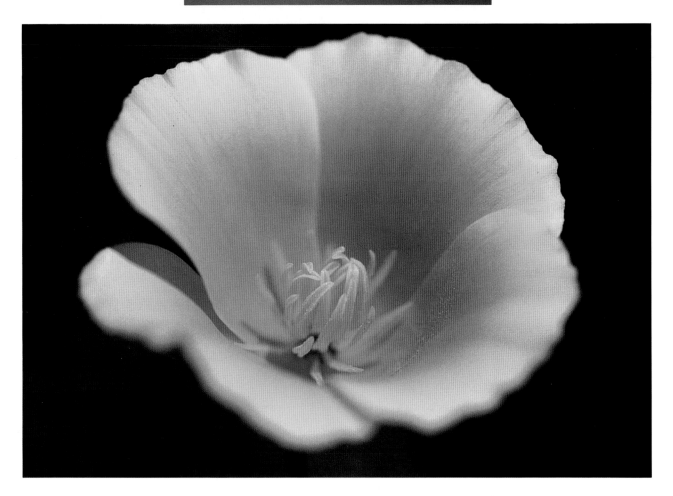

Defining the Horizon

Landscapes continue to be a popular subject for many photographers. A sunrise along the coast of Maine or a sunset on the sandy beaches of Maui is enticing; yet despite the beauty in such landscapes, good compositions seldom prevail. The reasons for this may be attributed to lens choice, point of view, or even the wrong time of day or season, but the real reason landscape pictures usually fail is because of a lack of emphasis. As in all good photographs, visually proclaiming your focus in the landscape is critical for a successful composition.

Most landscapes include horizons, and when a landscape is composed with the horizon line running through the middle of the frame, the viewer's interest is divided. A split horizon can be a classic mistake, one made by many amateur photographers. Unless one part of the scene has more weight—whether it be the sun and sky or the sea and land below—the viewer will respond with ambivalence to the indecision expressed in the picture. If you haven't made a choice about what is important in your picture, how can you expect the viewer to know what it is that you mean to say?

The artists of ancient Greece developed a solution for achieving balance and emphasis in landscape compositions, a technique that later became popular with the artists of the Middle Ages and today is often called the rule of thirds. This theory of art suggests that using a high or low horizon line vitalizes landscape compositions. When you analyze the rule of third's effect on landscape pictures, it is hard to argue against the idea. When the emphasis is placed in the top two-thirds or bottom two-thirds of the frame, the viewer is better directed toward the subjects you've decided are most important in the scene.

Applying the rule of thirds to your landscapes is simply a matter of deciding what part of the scene should carry the most weight. Think of the rule of thirds as dividing space into two horizontal bars. One will be approximately twice as thick as the other. Because your response to a subject area's importance is based on its size, you'll naturally assign greater value to the thicker bar. If a picture's visual interest is stronger below the horizon line, then a high horizon-line placement is desirable. Putting the horizon low in the frame is suitable for pictures whose visual interest is greatest above the horizon line—when, for example, you want to focus on something in the sky.

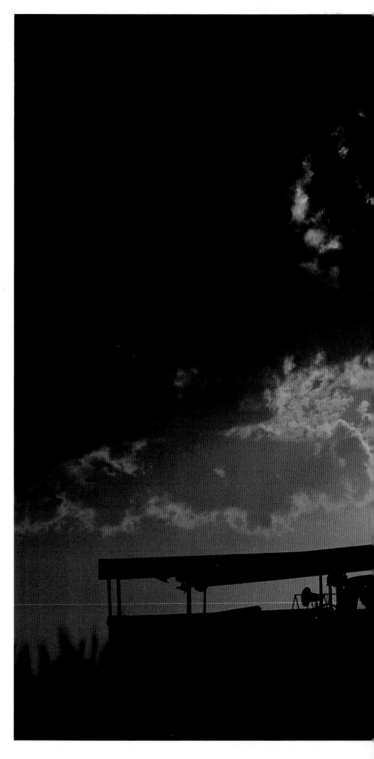

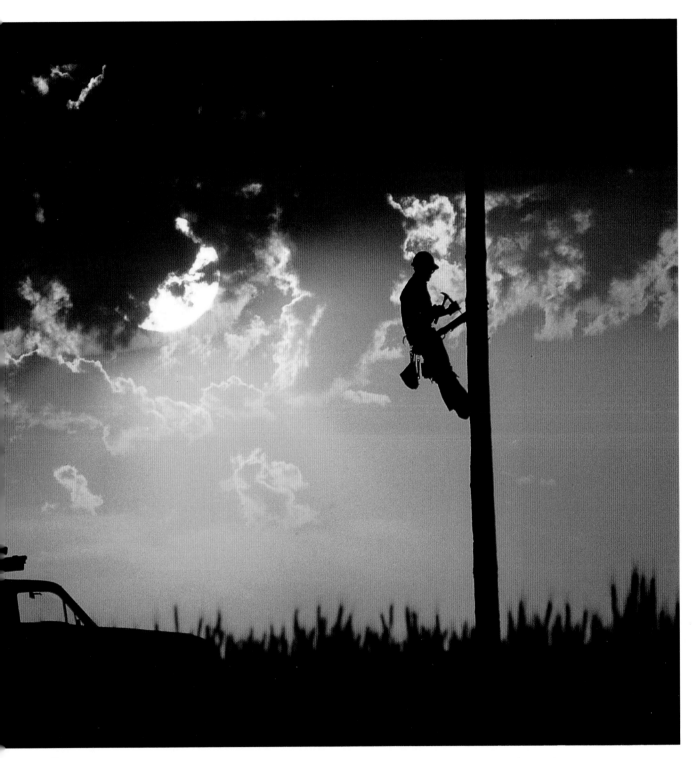

I had been working on assignment for a utility company for several days and had been staging compositions to illustrate the daily routines of the company's linemen. The final day of shooting took place on a country road in eastern Washington. Because the lineman, the pole, and the truck were all well above the horizon, choosing a low horizon line was the obvious way to showcase my subject interest. I used my 400mm lens because its vision reduces perspective and therefore put even greater emphasis on the silhouetted shapes.

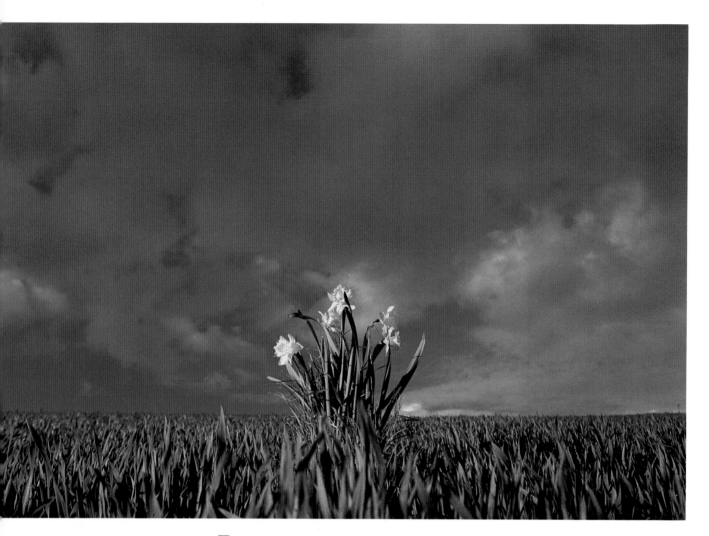

Following the winter purchase of my farm, my first spring there brought forth many surprises. One was discovering a single clump of daffodils in a nearby wheat field. In sharp contrast to the surrounding field of green the bright yellow flowers looked proud and boastful.

◆ Carefully stepping between rows of spring wheat to approach the flowers, I chose to photograph them from a low viewpoint with my 24mm wide-angle lens. The low horizon line, combined with the sweeping vision of the wide angle, pushed the flowers against the vast sky and consequently emphasized their message: "Jump for joy for spring has sprung!"

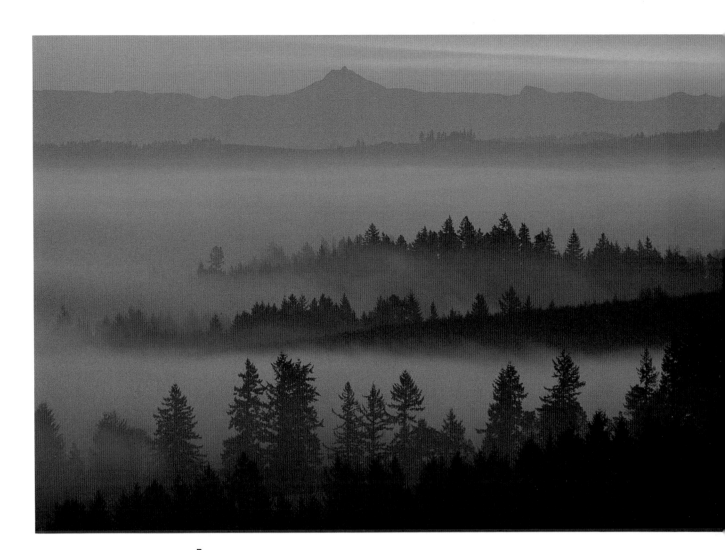

I love foggy days. Like fresh snowfall, fog brings a sense of newness to landscapes. High on a hill in Oregon's Willamette Valley, I watched the sun rise in a pastel pink sky while the trees below bobbed in a sea of fog. From this viewpoint I felt the scene's visual interest was greater below the horizon line. With my 200mm lens I framed the diagonally sloped hills and included only a fraction of the sky in the composition. Note how the subtle pink sky contrasts with the stillness and mystery of the trees.

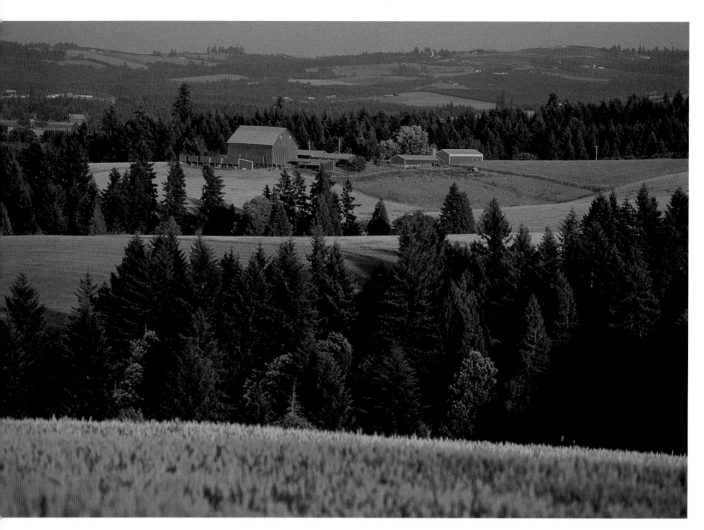

Six months later I had occasion to return to the same hilltop. I was on an assignment to photograph "a typical farmstead," and felt confident that the area's rolling fields of wheat, the trees, and this proverbial red farmstead would be the perfect an-swer. Using my 200mm lens on a tripod, I placed the emphasis in the pic-ture on the landscape be-low the horizon by including only a fraction of the sky. Notice, however, how the sky adds depth and perspective to this composition.

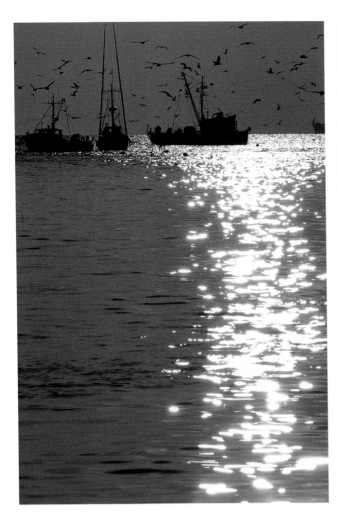
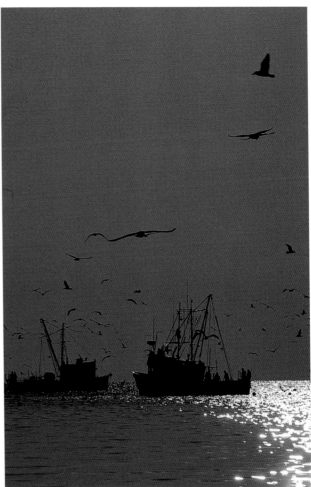

Sometimes a high or low horizon can work equally well. This usually happens when the scene simultaneously offers the same amount of interest above and below the horizon line. ◆ One such instance occurred while I was shooting near San Francisco at China Basin. Within several minutes of sunrise the commercial fishermen began to head out to sea. Their boats, the seagulls in the air, and the long, broad line of golden sunlight on the water created interest both above and below the horizon line. ◆ Both of these compositions work, but notice that the low horizon line on the right makes the boats appear closer. This is because we automatically assume that the low objects in a picture frame are closer to us. In addition, the broad vertical line of golden sunlight in the other composition creates an impression of depth and distance.

Vertical Versus Horizontal

Perhaps it is because a camera is more comfortable to hold in the horizontal position, or perhaps it is because the viewfinder's information is easier to read when the camera is horizontal—whatever the reason, many photographers suffer from "horizontalitis," or an addiction to the horizontal frame. It's not that using this format is bad, but the opportunities for vertical compositions are just as numerous and shouldn't be overlooked. Imagine both frames as hollow rectangles, and look at them side by side. If you could lie down inside either one, which would you choose? The horizontal rectangle, no doubt, since it offers more room to stretch out and relax. Conversely, if you were to stand up inside either one, which would you choose? The vertical rectangle, of course, since it offers more headroom.

In terms of emotion, the horizontal frame evokes calm feelings of tranquility just as a horizontal line does. In contrast, the vertical frame evokes feelings of pride and dignity. Quite often, subjects can be well composed in either format. Each conveys a different mood. I often find it critical to shoot a subject both ways since I market my work to a varied clientele. Some clients want only a vertical format—for instance, for magazine covers. No matter how wonderful my horizontal compositions are, they just won't work on most magazine covers.

Whenever you compose a picture, you should shoot in the format that calls the most attention to your subject. As you study each new opportunity, ask yourself whether the given subject could work equally well either way. There is no better time to decide than while you are at the picture site. After looking at the subject both ways, if you can't decide which looks better, take the picture both ways. One thing I've learned over the years is that film is very, very cheap compared to the trauma of having missed a wonderful shot.

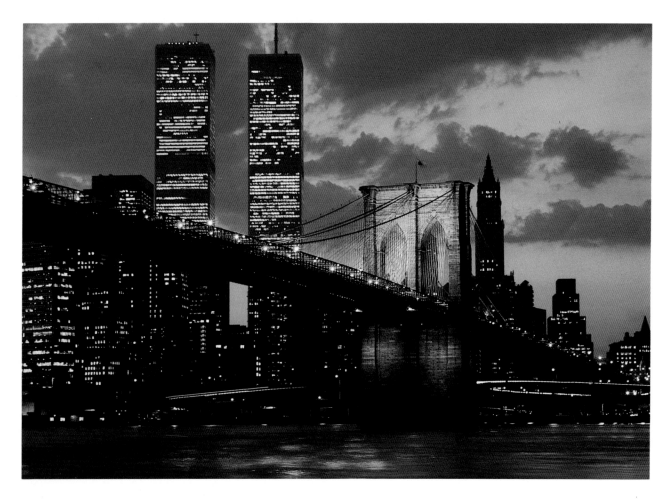

On the last day of a five-day assignment in New York City I was elated to hear that the weather forecast was calling for clear skies by nightfall. This came on the heels of four previous days of non-stop rain. I was determined to get a night shot of Lower Manhattan and the Brooklyn Bridge with a colorful sunset sky in the background. ◆ After finding an ideal vantage point in Brooklyn, I mounted my 105mm lens on my tripod and decided on an exposure time of 8 seconds at *f*/16. I first chose to frame the scene horizontally. Note the calm that prevails in the overall mood of this picture. Then I turned the tripod handles until the camera was in a vertical position. See how the mood of the city changes? Now the city skyline appears to be taller and prouder, an illusion created by your eyes having to travel a greater vertical distance in the photograph.

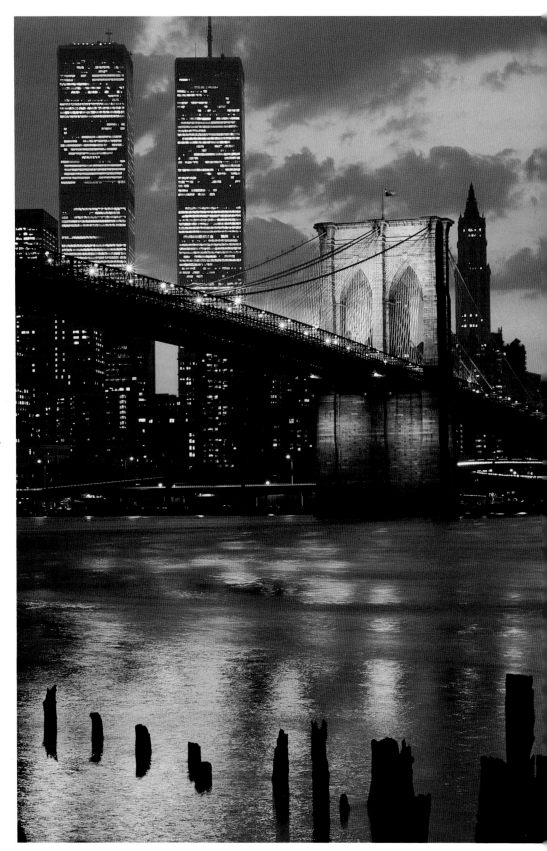

I have photographed many compositions of Mt. Hood from high up on the dirt and gravel roads that wind their way through the wheat country of north central Oregon. To the west the mountain sits ominously in the background. After a full day of shooting on assignment, I was resigned to heading back to my motel room and getting a good night of sleep. ◆ However, I was detoured by the light show in the western sky. Frantically searching for an unobstructed view of the mountain, I drove up to a high point and jumped from my car. Resting my 105mm lens and a firm pair of elbows on the hood of my car, I quickly fired off several frames before the colors of the sky faded. ◆ Notice how the horizontal composition evokes a calm, tranquil atmosphere while the vertical frame evokes feelings of strength and power because of the increased weight given to the sky. The mountain plays an important role in this composition, too, not as the main subject but as a visual resting place for the viewer's eye.

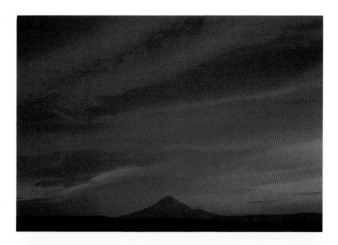

| LEARNING
TO SEE
CREATIVELY

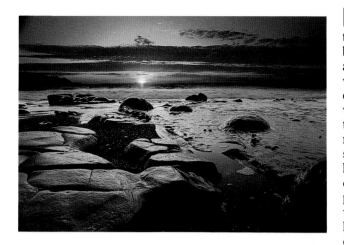

Imagine for a moment that the vertical sides of both these compositions are walls. Obviously, if you were to scale over the wall of the vertical frame, you would be much higher off the ground once you reached the top. This visual illusion of greater height is very popular with experienced landscape photographers, particularly when using the wide-angle lens. ◆ In the horizontal composition of a sunset at the beach, notice how I've abided by the rules and placed the horizon line in the top third of the frame since I felt the most interesting part of the picture fell below the horizon line. The rocks in the foreground help evoke a sense of depth and perspective. ◆ However, when the same subject is recomposed inside the vertical frame, the sense of depth and perspective is magnified. This is a very powerful illusion created by the eye traveling a greater distance from the bottom to the top of the picture. The smooth textured rock in the foreground was also calculated to stimulate viewer response—the pleasant smoothness reactivates the viewers' experiences with texture.

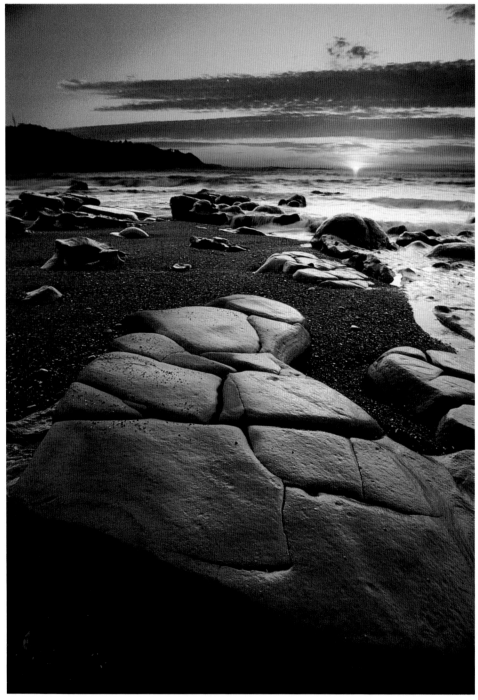

Skewing the Point of View

Tilting the camera so that it records your subjects on the diagonal is a way to introduce a feeling of speed, movement, and action to your compositions. As I've said earlier, a horizontal line suggests calm, a vertical line suggests pride, and a diagonal line suggests action. For instance, if you saw your house painter's ladder lying on your lawn, you'd either assume that he hadn't started painting or that he'd just finished for the day. If the ladder were resting diagonally against the building, you'd assume he was in the process of painting. Why? Because the ladder's diagonal line implies an uncompleted action. A plane taking off and moving diagonally toward the heavens is another good example. Once the plane reaches its cruising altitude, it levels off. If you've ever flown, you've experienced the tremendous power of the diagonal lift-off versus the calmer, quieter, horizontal cruising pattern of flight.

Many pictures in this book owe their impact to being composed on the diagonal. Regardless of whether I sought diagonal subjects or deliberately positioned the camera to record a strong diagonal line, these compositions are filled with action, growth, movement, or speed. If my photography is an outward expression of my psyche, as my peers have suggested, then I would hope that the same growth and speed reflected in so many of my compositions is also going on inside of me.

Graphic details pulled out of larger scenes generally make the best diagonal compositions. Purposely skewing the point of view seldom works in photographs of landscapes, entire buildings, or people; seeing the world presented on a tilt may lead the viewer to question the photographer's sobriety. But when it comes to isolating details, the opportunities for diagonal framing are plentiful.

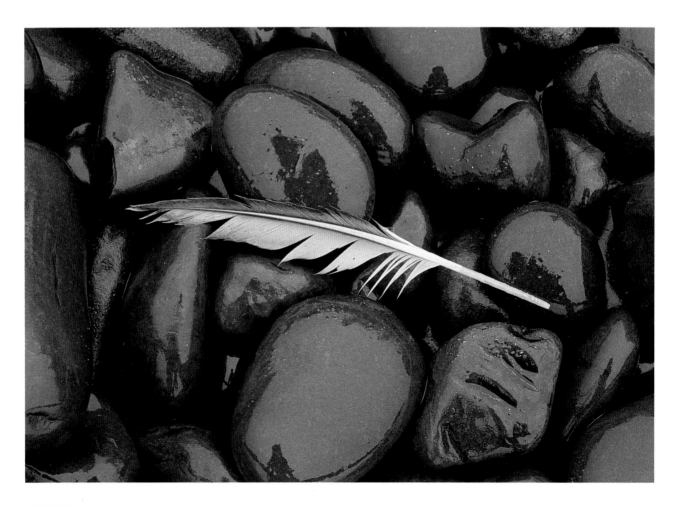

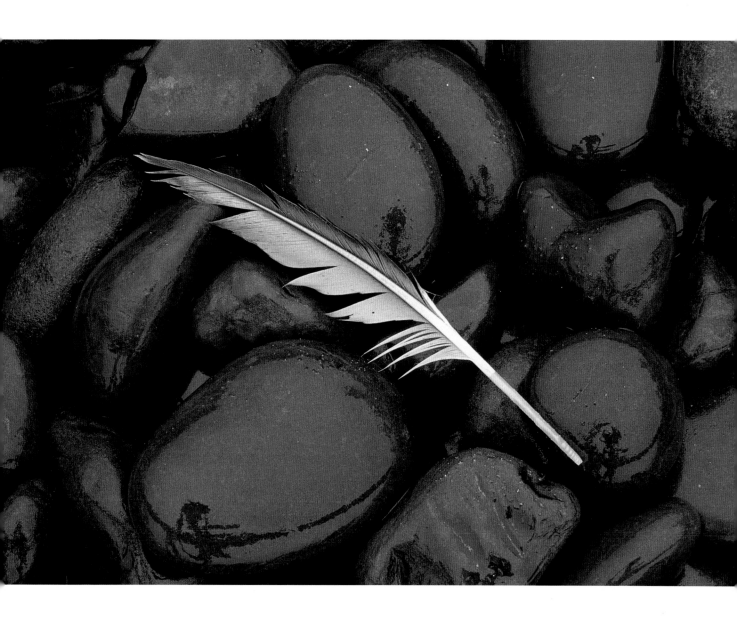

Along Oregon's beaches the shorelines provide unlimited studies of form, texture, and pattern. Several days of high winds and rain made the rocky shoreline of Indian Head Beach a resting place for countless feathers. I was struck by the contrast in textures: the soft, delicate feathers against hard rocks. ◆ With my 50mm normal lens I framed one feather against the rocks inside the horizontal frame. This composition looked lethargic, and I felt the need to bring the feather to life. A simple, diagonal shift in the camera's position created the desired effect by adding tension to the image.

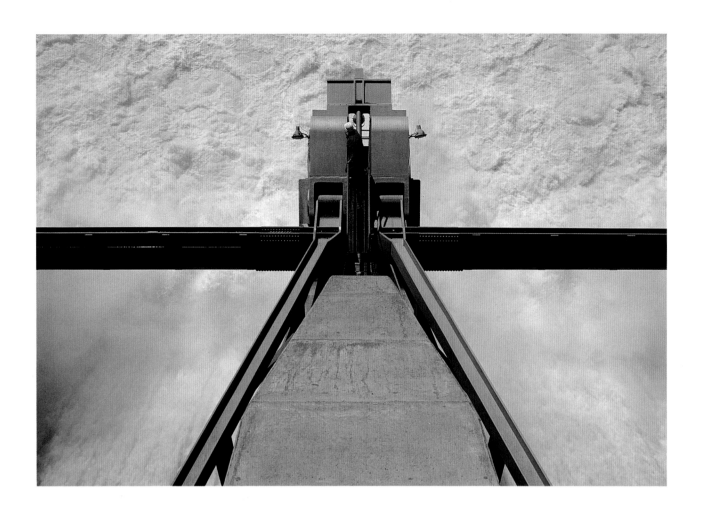

Choosing a viewpoint high above the spill gates of the John Day Dam in Oregon, I wanted to create a dizzying perspective. Leaning out over the edge of the catwalk and shooting straight down with my 24mm wide-angle lens, I was immediately struck by the strong horizontal bar crossing the frame. It had the force of a roadblock, bringing an abrupt halt to the drama of the composition. Without skipping a beat I broke through this barrier by turning the camera diagonally and made a dynamic image.

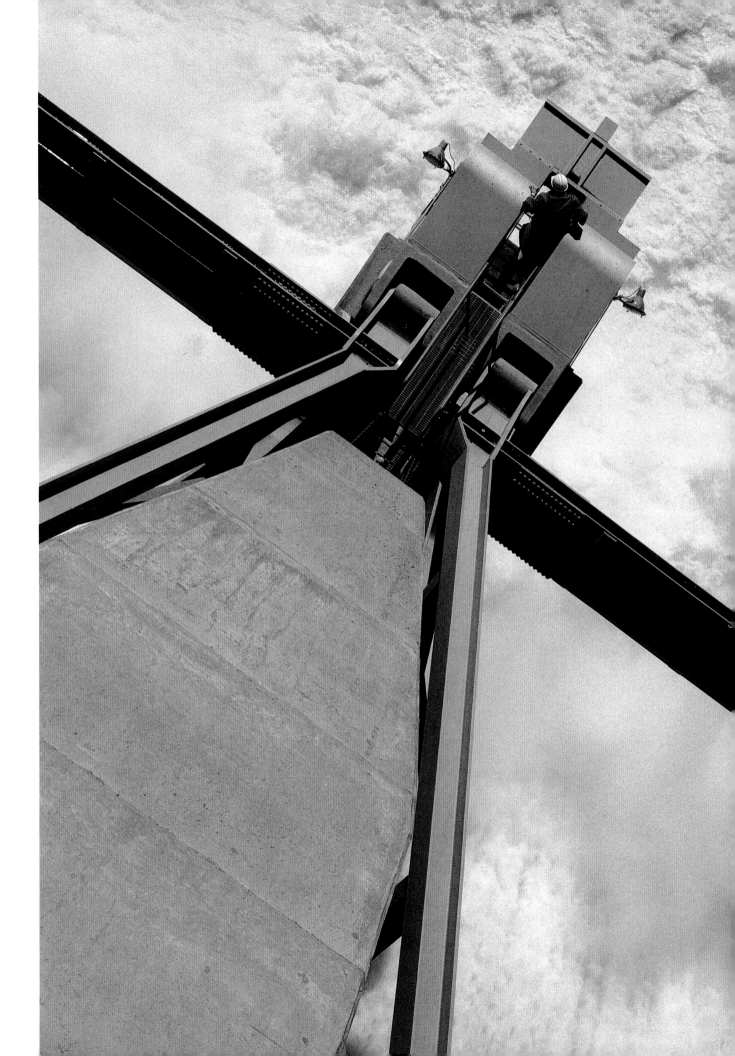

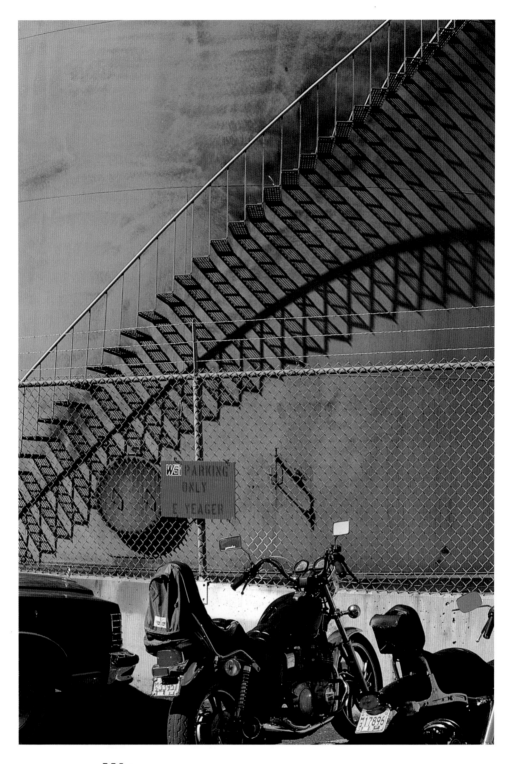

While I was shooting in an industrial area filled with oil storage tanks, my eyes became fixed on the natural diagonal flow of the stairway that leads to the top of the tank shown in the top picture. I became curious about what might happen if I straightened out the stairway with my camera; so I began looking at it on the diagonal through my 105mm lens. By composing only the steps and their shadows, I was able to make this abstract detail. Without seeing the larger scene, you might have difficulty identifying the stairs in the detail shot. This particular composition continues to be one of my favorites.

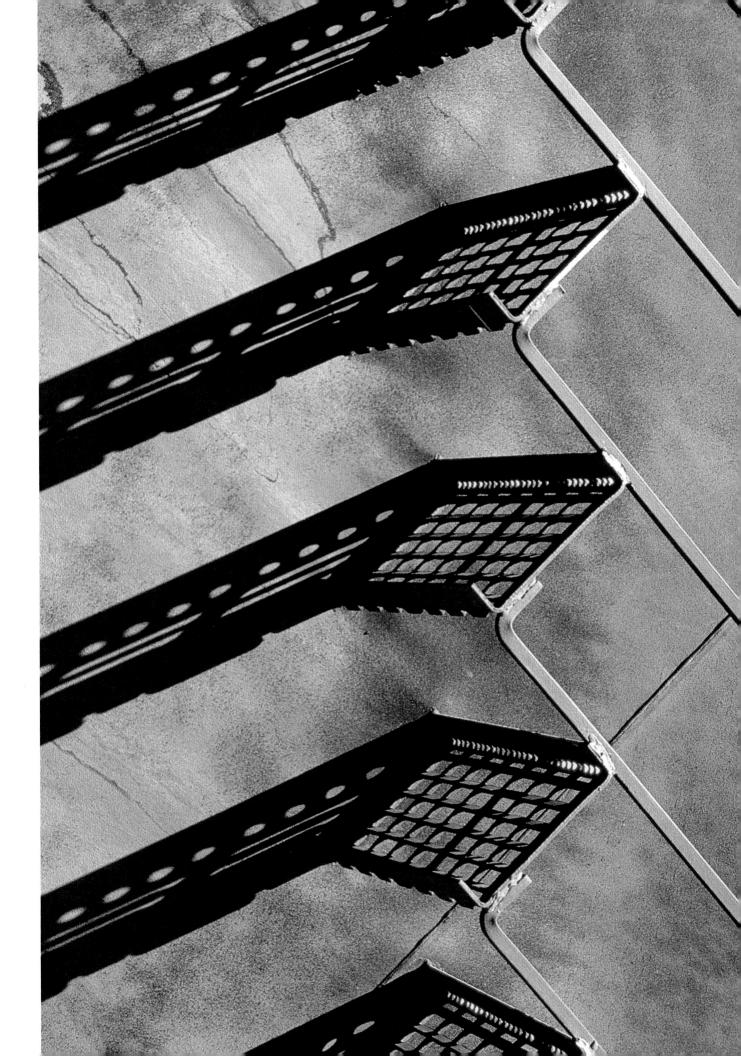

Framing the Image

One of the greatest clichés seen in landscape photography is the scene viewed through overhanging branches. It may be hackneyed, but it is still effective. Framing the image this way limits the field of view and calls attention to the subject. This is also one of the simplest ways to create perspective since it always brings a sense of depth to a composition. You can easily frame an image with telephoto lens by focusing through the foreground, thereby throwing it out of focus and directing the viewer's attention to the focused object further away from the camera. Of course, the foreground frame doesn't have to be out of focus; you may want it focused to sharply define the picture's edges.

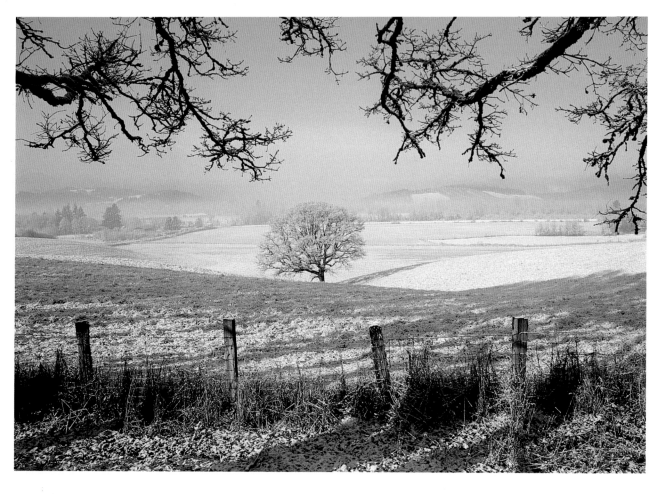

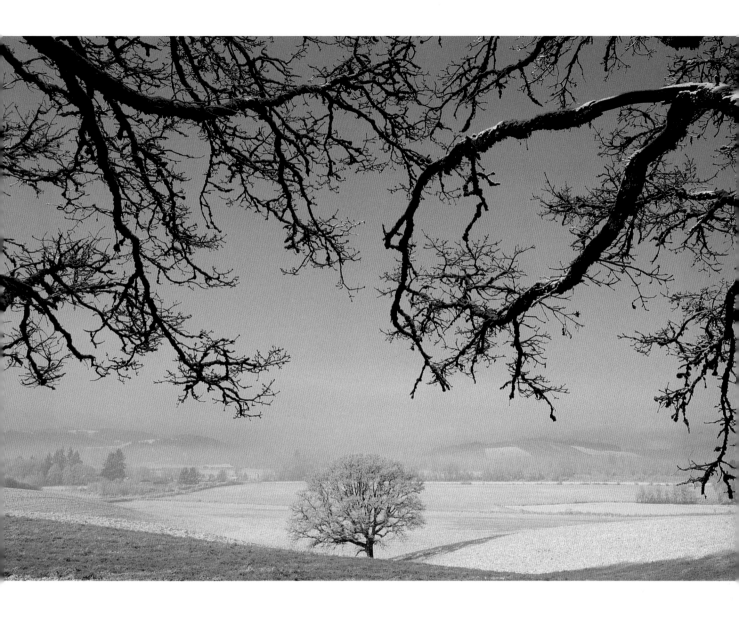

At the bottom of the hill near my house, a lone oak rules the pasture around it. Bordering this pasture on three sides are rows of other oak trees. Not until a winter snowfall did I notice this scene while driving to the grocery store. I always keep my cameras ready in the car; so I reached into the back seat and put my 24mm lens on my camera. Standing at the edge of the road, I shot these pic-tures. ◆ I wanted to place the emphasis on the lone oak in the pasture, but the strong horizontal line of the fence seemed to be a barrier. Raising my camera higher and walking to the edge of the fence, I was able to eliminate the fence and frame the dis-tant oak with the nearby branches of the foreground trees. Notice the powerful lines in this picture and how they direct the eye to my subject, the lone oak.

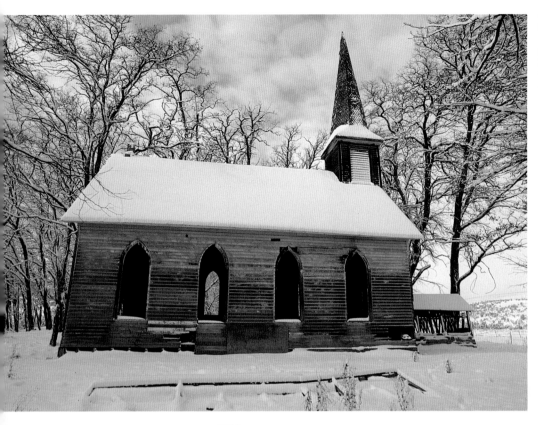

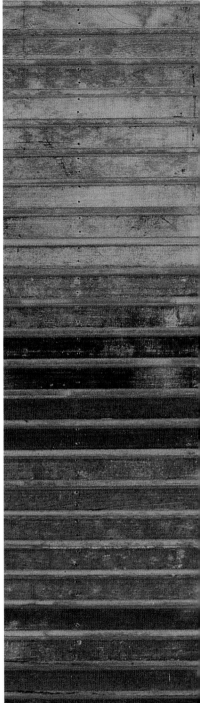

Wintertime in Oregon brings a stillness to the air that I find most enjoyable, particularly east of the Cascade Mountains. Sitting quietly in a grove of trees, the Old Locust Church harbors many opportunities for photographic exploration. As I walked across the church's snow-covered grounds, the crunch of ice and snow beneath my feet spooked a great horned owl off of his perch. ◆ Several minutes later, my eyes zeroed in on a window framing the shape of another window behind it and the snow-covered trees beyond the church. I mounted my 105mm lens on my tripod and set my aperture at *f*/22; then I adjusted the depth-of-field scale to assure sharpness throughout the image. Because the second window was in open shade, its shape recorded as black since I was exposing for the lighted exterior, including the trees. The black-shaped window creates an even greater sense of depth than framing usually achieves because we generally experience black as being a fathomless space.

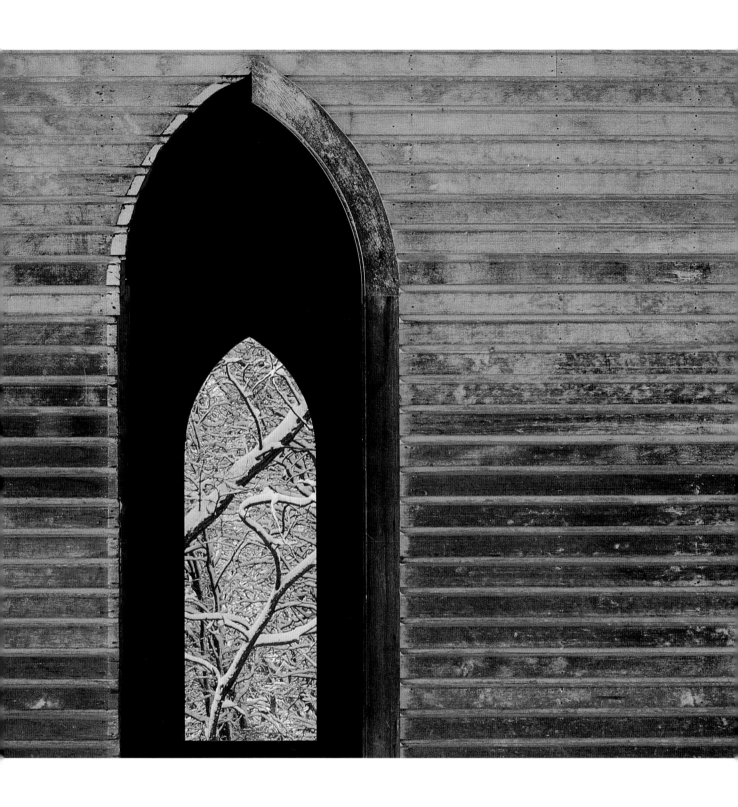

Silhouetting the Subject

Perhaps nothing is more satisfying to the amateur photographer than producing a well-composed silhouette. A stark, barely defined shape frees the viewer's imagination to run wild without interference from texture or color. Silhouettes commonly occur when a subject is backlit and the camera's exposure is set exclusively for the backlight. These conditions ensure that all the objects in front of the backlight will be rendered as silhouettes.

Silhouettes may be easy to create, but they end up looking dismal on film if they merge together. In the business world two companies merge together and become one, but what is good for business is seldom good for silhouettes. You can avoid embarrassing mergers by thinking like an exposure meter. The human eye can cope with vast ranges of light and dark simultaneously. On the other hand, your camera's exposure meter and your film are limited to recording a much narrower range of lighting zones. When their range of light and shadow exceeds plus or minus two stops, something in your picture has to give. Either you'll end up with perfectly exposed shadows and washed out highlights, or you'll end up with perfectly exposed highlights and severely underexposed or black shadows.

So as you look through the viewfinder, remind yourself that all the objects in front of the backlight are going to become black shapes if your exposure is for the strong backlight, and make sure that from your vantage point, none of these objects overlap. Otherwise, they'll create unsightly mergers between various silhouetted subjects in the final picture. Shutting off your brain's interpretation of a given lighting situation and seeing like an exposure meter will enable you to successfully visualize how your silhouetted compositions will appear on film.

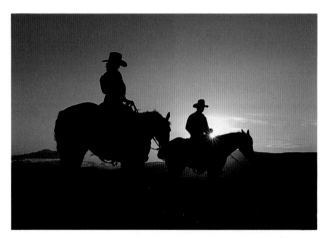 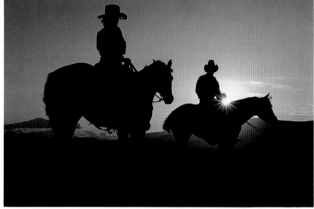

As I stood in this open field, anxious to shoot a couple of Oregon cowboys, I could see that my camera position was too high and would cause the horses and riders to merge with the faraway hills. Shifting to a lower position, I was able to push the riders you see in these two pictures up above the distant horizon, which showcased them against a clean background. ◆ Though my eyes told me that the horses were tan and the riders were wearing blue jeans and colorful flannel shirts, I reminded myself that they would become black shapes on film since my exposure was for the bright sky and sun. Confident that I was ready, I began to shoot, but after two shots I realized the head of the horse closest to me was merging with the other horse's rear end. To correct this embarrassing merger I moved in closer and got down a bit lower, which corrected the awkward perspective.

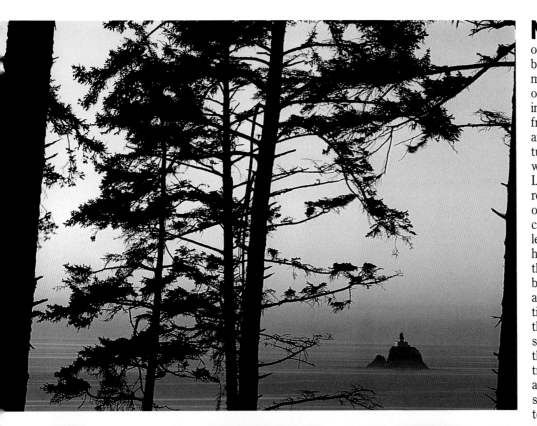

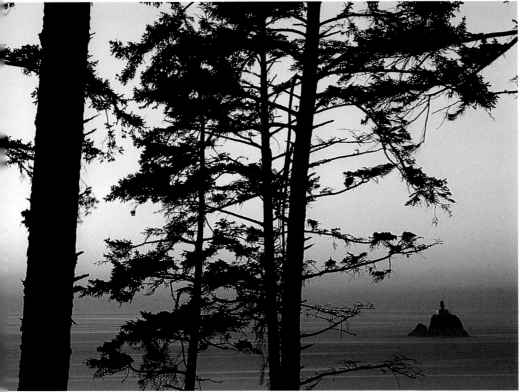

Not as obvious to everyone as the last example but just as bothersome to me are the mergers that occur along the edges or in the corners of the frame. A few minutes after shooting a sunset, I turned my attention towards Tillamook Head Lighthouse. It sits atop a rock island several miles off the northern Oregon coast. Using my 200mm lens, I framed the lighthouse with some trees in the foreground, which brought a sense of scale and depth to the composition. I set my exposure for the strong backlight of the sunset sky, ensuring that the green, moss-covered tree trunks would record as stark, silhouetted shapes on film. ◆ In the top picture, however, notice the tree intruding on the right edge of the frame. In my haste to record the scene I failed to see what I consider a merger. I find the tension this intrusion creates very disturbing. It looks as if the tree is trying to "crash the party" or "made a mad dash for the elevator but got caught in the closing doors." Basically, the tree's presence makes the composition look indecisive and sloppy. By shifting my viewpoint just a little bit to the left, I was able to eliminate the intrusion.
◆ Get in the habit of running your eyes along all four edges of the frame *before* you press the shutter. Because most landscape compositions don't require split-second responses, take a few extra moments and really look at what your viewfinder is showing you. The worst time to discover mergers or intrusions is after your film has been processed.

Breaking the Rules

"Centering your subject creates a static feeling and makes the viewer feel tense. Don't place your horizon line through the middle of the frame because you end up with a composition that lacks emphasis. And whatever you do, always remember to fill the frame with your subject!" Like many other rules in life, these rules of composition are intended to keep you on the straight and narrow, but adhering to them doesn't ensure great photography. Follow the rules and you'll make pleasant compositions; however, just as a wanderer veers off a well-worn path in the woods and rejoices upon discovering a hidden waterfall, you can make rewarding discoveries if you are willing to break the rules.

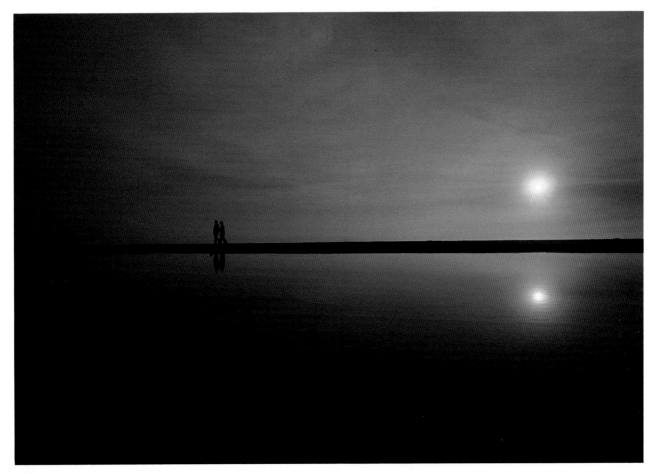

Many camera clubs seem bent on criticizing landscape compositions where the horizon line splits the middle of the frame. For authority, they quote the rule that says, "Without a high or low horizon line, the viewer can't tell what part of the scene carries the most weight." When you encounter mirroring situations such as this one, I suggest you forget this rule and start deliberately exploring opportunities to split the frame in two.

◆ Tidal pools are often left behind low tide along the central Oregon coast. Crawling on my belly to the edge of one large pool, I fired off several frames with my 24mm lens before this passing couple exited from my viewfinder. Rather than dividing the pictures interest, I think you'll agree that putting the horizon in the center of the picture doubles its impact. Also, on closer inspection you'll see that the areas above and below the horizon line both follow the rule of thirds.

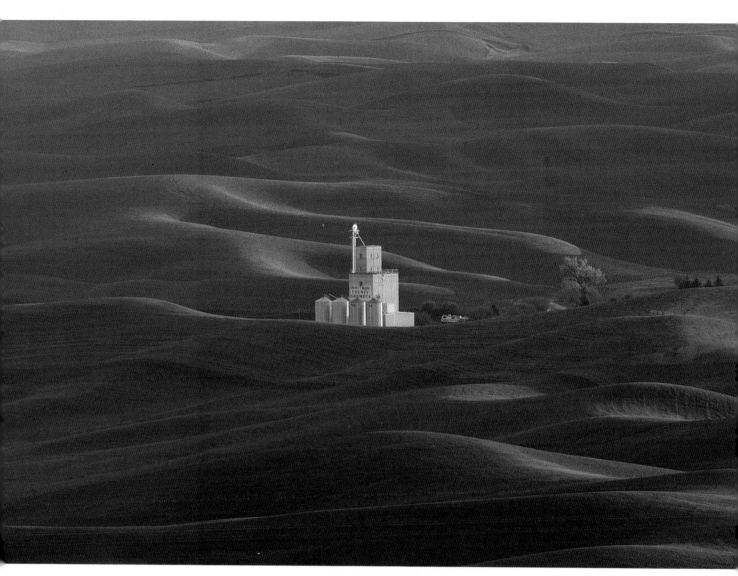

Another common criticism is directed at pictures that suffer from the bull's-eye effect: a composition whose key subject is dead centered, imparting a static feeling. However, this picture is evidence that this kind of 'mistake' can be made to work for you. Returning to the Palouse Country in eastern Washington, I purposely found the same rolling fields and grain elevator I had shot six months earlier. Using my 50–300mm zoom lens set at the 300mm focal length, I framed the grain elevators smack dab in the middle of the frame. So why does this work here? The rolling hill's curvilinear lines continually lead the eye on a quiet journey, and this simple, constant movement keeps the picture from feeling anything but static. When the eye gets tired, it can go to the center and rest upon the stable shapes of the grain elevators.

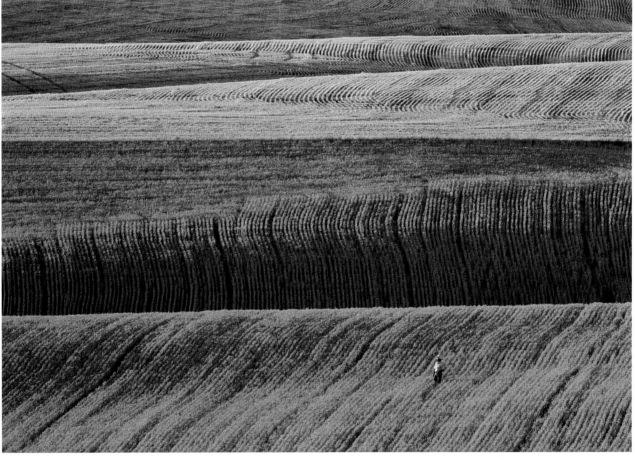

All three of these pictures have one thing in common. Their tiny subjects—the oak, the farmer, and two workers—clearly grab and hold the viewer's attention. But how can this be when they don't even come close to filling the frame?

◆ The answer lies in a basic law of visual perception. The smaller a subject is in relation to surrounding contrasts or shapes, the more unusual it appears. And the more unusual or isolated a subject is, the more it stands out.

◆ Upon closer inspection you can see that each frame is, in fact, filled to the brim with contrasting tones, textures, and shapes. This allowed the dark-colored oak to stand out in an otherwise monochromatic landscape. With my 24mm lens raised high I was able to record enough contrasting tones to push the oak even farther back in the frame, which diminished its size even more. ◆ Because the farmer's shape jumps out in contrast to the surrounding tones and textures of the rolling fields of wheat, he clearly gets the viewer's attention. Using my 400mm lens, I was able to reduce the depth of field and thereby stack the hills of wheat in this picture. ◆ I experimented with my 105mm lens and my point of view to record this pattern of curvilinear shapes. They are actually water mains six feet in diameter. Their shapes stand in marked contrast to those of the humans astride them.

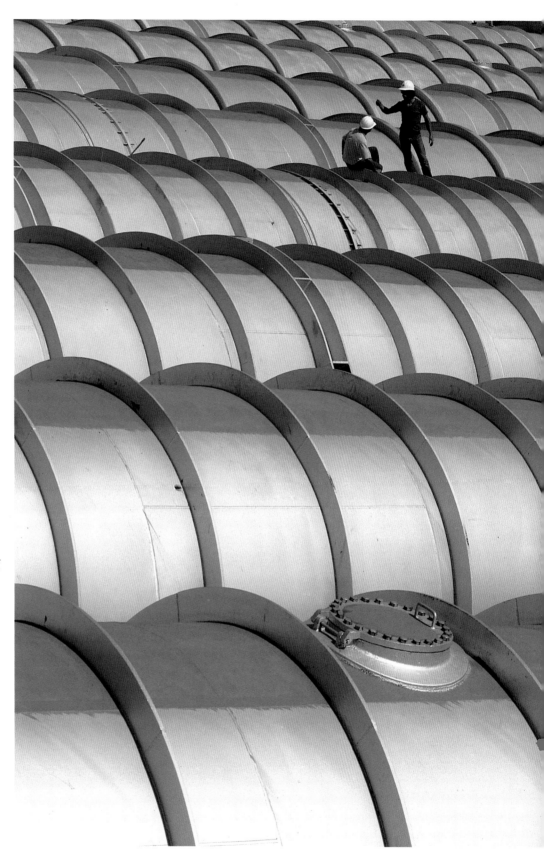

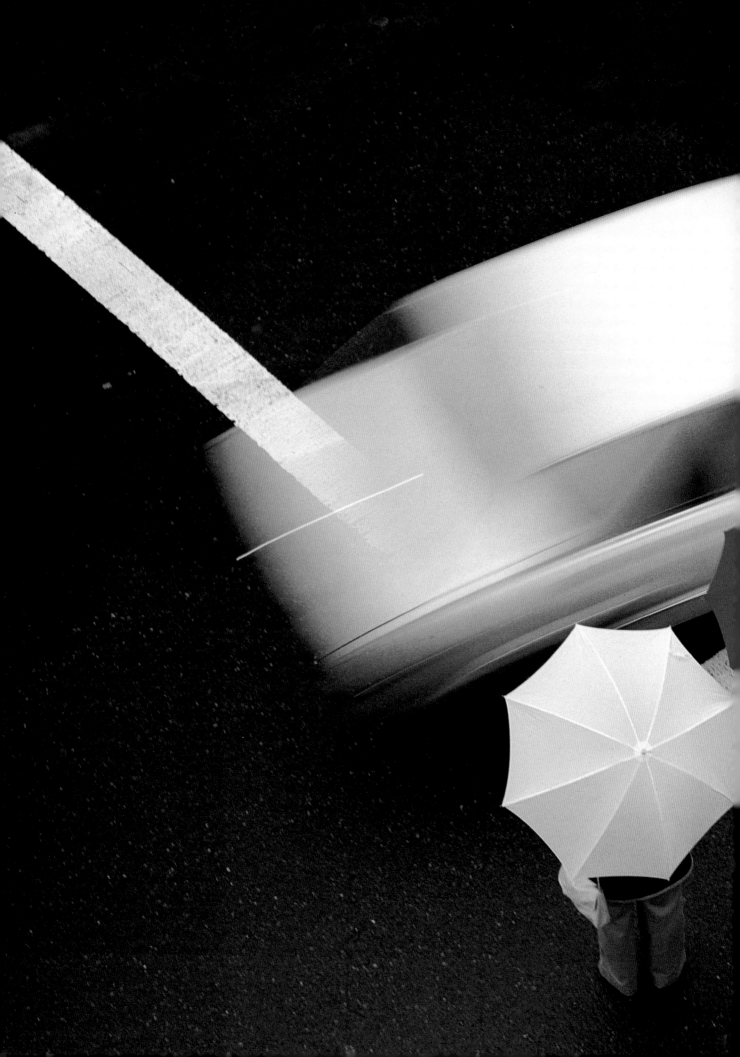

UNDERSTANDING YOUR EXPOSURE OPTIONS

More than a dozen kinds of film are currently available for 35mm cameras. Having so many choices has lead to a lot of confusion about which films are best for action, for low-light situations, for closeups, and for portraits. Films with speeds between ISO 50 and ISO 100 are fast enough to handle most of your picture-taking needs and unlike their faster counterparts (ISO 200–1600) offer rich color, fine grain, and improved sharpness.

Some photographers argue against using slower films because they resent "dragging a tripod" with them everywhere they go. I've discovered that photographers who don't want to use a tripod are usually the least successful at composing and taking good pictures. Shooting with a tripod will increase your photographic opportunities a hundred-fold, so why argue against it? Without a tripod you can't: shoot in pre-dawn light or after the sun goes down; shoot exposures longer than 1/15 sec.; successfully use long telephoto lenses; shoot extreme closeups at small lens openings; record straight horizon lines; and the list goes on and on. Not one single photograph in this book was exposed on a film faster than ISO 64, and only nine photographs were taken without my tripod.

One of photography's challenges is to strike the correct balance between the shutter speed and the aperture. A range of aperture/shutter-speed combinations exists in any given lighting situation. In terms of the volume of light that reaches the film, $f/8$ at 1/125 sec. is the same exposure as $f/5.6$ at a 1/250 sec. or $f/11$ at a 1/60 sec. This doesn't mean you should randomly pick and choose your exposure combinations. The creative use of shutter speeds and f-stops is not simply a matter of multiple choice. If you use a shutter speed that is too slow, you can't freeze action. A shutter speed that is too fast inhibits the ability to imply action. If you use an aperture opening that is too large, you'll lose precious depth of field, but an aperture opening that is too small prevents you from being able to selectively focus. As you can see, your choice of f-stop and shutter speed should depend solely on the creative effect you want.

I found another opportunity to pan my camera for movement when one of my horses was in a spirited mood, running almost wildly in the pasture. First I set my shutter speed at 1/60 sec., and then I adjusted the aperture until the correct exposure was indicated. As the horse ran by parallel to me, I moved the camera along with him in the same direction. This kept him sharp while rendering the background as a series of streaked blurs. A storm was brewing, but luckily, a window opened up in the clouds, and light happened to shine down right on the horse while I was taking the picture.

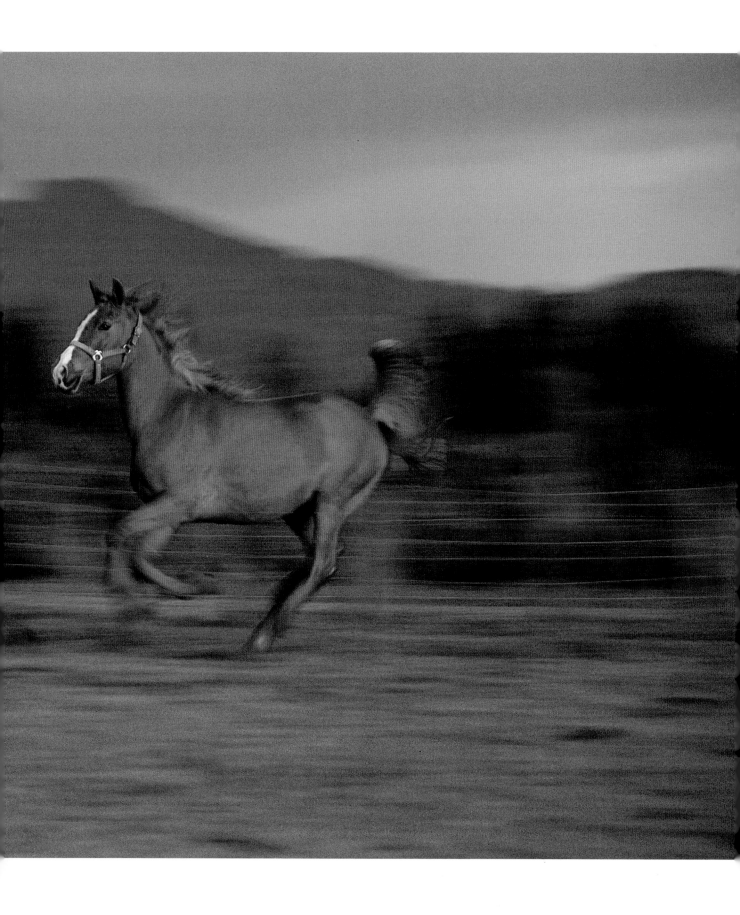

Shutter Speed

How well do you see motion? As a component of the visible, physical world, motion is a wonderful subject for still photography, even though you can only record it symbolically in a nonmoving image. Photographers are usually concerned with freezing motion and stopping it cold with a very fast shutter speed to produce a razor-sharp image. However, this is not the only way to record motion; indeed, it is sometimes the least interesting. Blurring the subject or the background may be a more effective way to say something about the impact of movement. Using a slow shutter speed to record a fast moving subject will render a trail of subject images across the film, and this blur will contrast nicely with the rest of the sharply focused picture. Blurring the background and keeping the subject sharp is a little more tricky, but it is a powerful way to evoke and isolate the subject's own perspective and experience. (Panning is the technique for doing this—you move the camera along with your subject at the same rate of speed it is moving, and expose it at the same time.)

If your subject doesn't require or lend itself to motion-filled opportunities, then finding the right aperture should always be your first concern, and the shutter speed should be chosen solely for the right exposure. Depth of field depends on aperture alone, which gives it precedence over shutter speed unless movement is your subject.

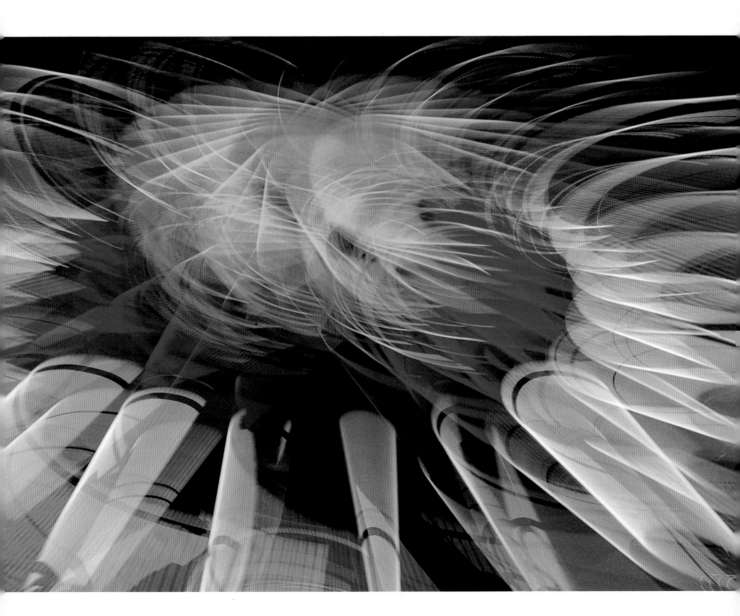

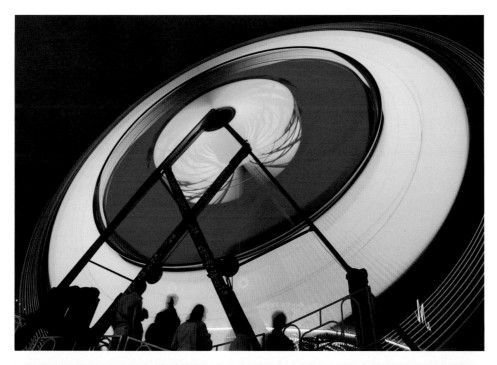

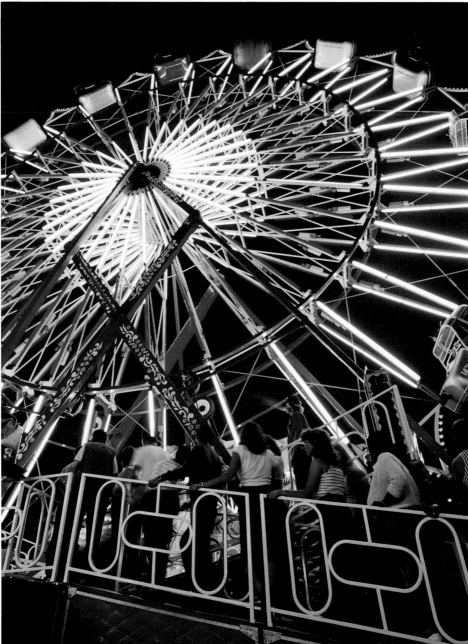

Amusement parks continue to be among my favorite subjects. Colors abound there and motion-filled rides are everywhere—splendid subject matter for capturing abstract images. You might feel inclined to choose a high-speed film with an ISO of 400 or 1000 to cope with low-light situations, such as the one in these pictures; then you could choose the fastest shutter speed possible and achieve a clear image like the bottom picture of a ferris wheel and the people waiting in line for their turn on the ride. ◆ But what if you used a slow–to–medium-speed film, such as ISO 50, 64, or 100, put your camera on a tripod, and recorded the motion of the ride instead? That is exactly what I did. Angling my 24mm lens upward, I set my shutter speed at one second and then adjusted my aperture until the correct exposure was indicated. Once the ride reached its maximum speed, I fired off several frames and recorded the colorful, flying-saucer shape in the top picture. ◆ Using the same exposure, I removed the camera from the tripod and panned the camera in the same direction as the moving ferris wheel. The resulting abstract image on the far left looks like bursting fireworks.

Aperture

Most photographers shoot landscapes, closeups, and people, all subjects where using the right *f*-stop spells the difference between success or failure. Generally speaking, there are three creative categories of apertures. The first category is used to shoot story-telling compositions. Most landscapes reveal a great deal of material, from the immediate foreground to the distant horizon. Often it is paramount that all this information record sharply on film, which is why I call *f*/16, *f*/22, and *f*/32 the "story-telling" apertures. On the other end of the aperture ring you'll find smaller numbers and bigger openings: *f*/2.8, *f*/4, and *f*/5.6. I refer to these as "singular-theme" apertures. When you want to limit your depth of field to focus on a single theme or subject and when you use selective focus, you'll need to call upon these wider apertures. The telephoto lens is a good tool for singular-theme compositions because its narrow angle of view helps to delete superfluous material from the image.

Finally, there are the "who-cares" apertures: *f*/8 and *f*/11. Who cares what *f*-stop you use when shooting straight down on frost-covered leaves? Who cares what *f*-stop is right for photographing someone standing up against a brick wall? In both cases the area of focus begins and ends with the subject. Depth of field is not like x-rays; it can't possibly go into the ground and make the worms sharp or pierce the brick wall and show the wooden studs behind it. In such situations, the reason I use *f*/8 or *f*/11 instead of other apertures is that *f*/8 and *f*/11 are the critical apertures—either provides amazing optical sharpness.

When composing story-telling pictures, beginners often wonder how it is possible to make everything from the immediate foreground to the distant horizon sharp. Well, it doesn't just depend on using a small lens opening. First, you must decide at what point you want sharpness to begin in the foreground. I favor sharpness in the immediate foreground, the foreground right at my feet. Because the wide-angle lens' wide, sweeping vision begins in the immediate foreground and travels to the distant horizon, I use it most often for story-telling pictures. But the question of where to focus still remains. I don't! Instead, I always preset my focus via the depth-of-field scale. I set my aperture at *f*/22 and align the distances I want sharp between the two hash marks on the lens, knowing that once I press the shutter, the area indicated between these hash marks will be sharp in the final picture.

Once beginners are made aware of this technique, they invariably question its validity since when they look through the viewfinder at a composition, everything still appears fuzzy. That is because all of today's 35mm SLRs offer wide-open viewing. This means that even though your aperture may be set at a much smaller lens opening—for instance, *f*/8, *f*/16 or *f*/32—you are still viewing the scene through a wide-open aperture, the bait that hooks you into thinking that "what you see is what you get." Believe me, using the depth-of-field scale is the only way to control the area of sharpness in your pictures when you want maximum depth of field. Make a habit of referring to it.

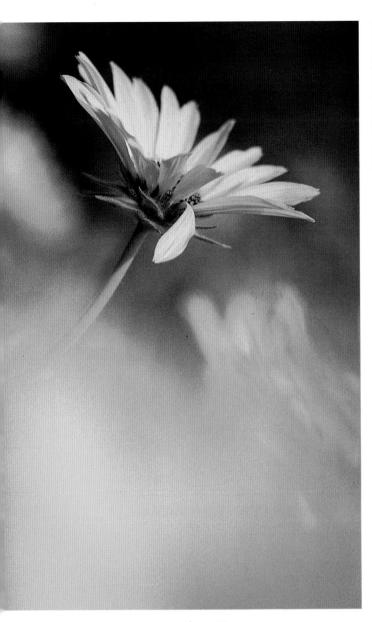

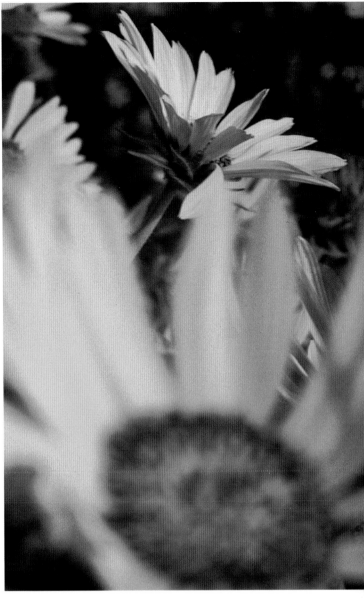

Across the hillsides in the Hood River Valley of Oregon the deep yellow flowers of the balsam root appear every spring. Such vivid color makes them a welcome relief following the long, dark days of winter. ◆ Moving among the flowers with my 200mm lens, I selectively focused upon a single bloom surrounded by a wash of out-of-focus color. But just because I saw this image in my viewfinder was no guarantee that I would record it on film. The only assurance of recording a singular-theme composition is to use a singular-theme aperture: *f*/2.8, *f*/4, or *f*/5.6.

◆ The picture on the left is a successful composition because I deliberately chose *f*/5.6, a singular-theme aperture. The righthand photograph, however, is the result of a story-telling aperture, *f*/16. It produced too much depth of field and a cluttered composition. Simply put, when you have a big story to tell, use the big *f*-stop numbers. When you have a very short story to tell, use the small *f*-stop numbers.

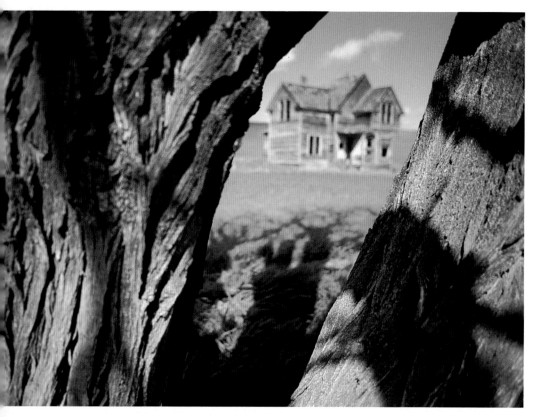

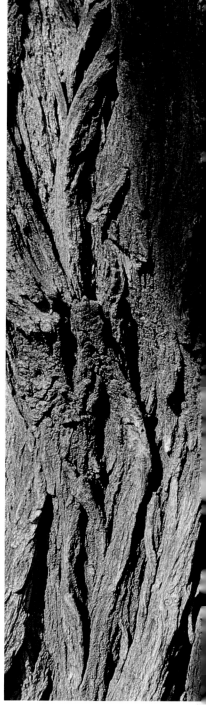

Being somewhat of a history buff, I'm always elated to discover an abandoned farmstead. One caught my eye near The Dalles, Oregon. After careful searching, I felt I could best tell the story of this old building by creating a foreground frame from an old locust tree. The rough texture of the tree's bark and its looming shadow is dramatic and invites viewer participation. I mounted my 24mm lens on a tripod and set my aperture at f/22; then I preset my focus according to the depth-of-field scale, so that everything from two feet to infinity would be sharp on film. Finally, I adjusted my shutter speed until a correct exposure was indicated. ◆ In the top photograph the building appears horribly out of focus. This is how the scene looked once I preset my focus. If you were taking this picture, at this point you might feel inclined to refocus the scene until the farmstead appeared sharp to your eye. But please, avoid this temptation in your own work. Simply remind yourself that what the viewfinder shows you is the product of wide-open metering. Once you've pressed the shutter, the lens will stop down to f/22, and objects will be rendered sharp as the depth-of-field scale promises. The other picture illustrates that without any refocusing effort on my part, sharpness did in fact occur throughout the scene.

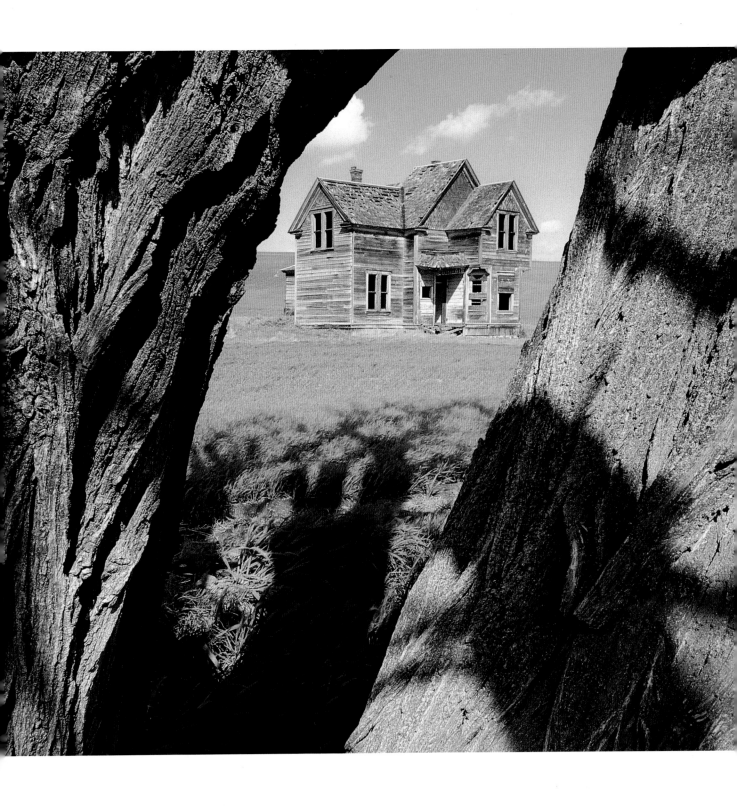

THE MAGIC
OF AVAILABLE
LIGHT

Light is constantly changing as the sun's position shifts throughout the day. The time of day you choose to shoot and your position vis-à-vis the sun determines a lot about how your subject will appear on film—hard or soft edged, in warm or cool tones, and displaying vivid details or glaring contrasts. Light has three important characteristics: brightness, color, and direction. All three undergo varying degrees of intensity depending on the time of day, and each affects the mood created by the light in any given scene. Careful study of these three attributes will enable you to take advantage of the powerful roles they play in establishing a photograph's emotional tone.

Paying attention to light and how it affects your subject's appearance is so important it can't be overstated. Photographers who don't understand or appreciate the impact that different kinds of light have on a scene usually complain about the lack of emotional response people have to their pictures. Of course, often you do pay a price for literally presenting your subjects in the best light possible. Arriving at a location long before the birds begin to sing may seem a bit crazy. Hanging out in a hot desert or on a mountain top in sub-zero temperatures to capture a special kind of light takes commitment. But when you spread your slides across a light table or look at your prints, you'll be glad you made the extra effort.

Whenever I arrive someplace new to take photographs, I'm anxious to get my bearings. I've had great success by visiting tourist shops in airports and bus stations where I buy postcards that show photographs of local attractions; then I immediately find a cab driver, show him or her the cards, and ask if the pictures were taken facing north, south, east, or west. Once I have my bearings, I spend the midday hours looking for fresh points of view of these same locales. If everything goes as planned, I will then shoot them in the late afternoon or early morning light. Scouting a location for good camera positions before you start shooting takes dedication, but it also eliminates surprises. There is nothing worse than being caught off guard in a valley fifteen minutes before sunset while the blazing sun drops behind a mountain top. The trouble is, you didn't have a shooting plan, so now you're trapped without a vantage point in the wrong spot. If you had mapped out a shooting plan in advance, you would be perched high on a ridge, capturing the last light on film.

The more experience you get working on location with available light, the better your photographs will be. You'll learn to assess a subject's potential under various lighting conditions, regardless of the light in which you initially see it. Daily practice with your camera—changing points of view, switching lenses, and working with different kinds of light—will culminate in a tremendous visual awareness and bring you closer to learning to see creatively.

Arriving early one morning at my brother's farm, I found my sister-in-law Amy tending to the many chores that her farm life demands. I decided to photograph her to illustrate a story idea I had about working women on the farm. ◆ First I photographed her in open shade, creating a composition that lacked vivid color. As you can see, her skin tone appears to be quite pale. Portraits seldom have emotional appeal when photographed in open shade. Shadows re-

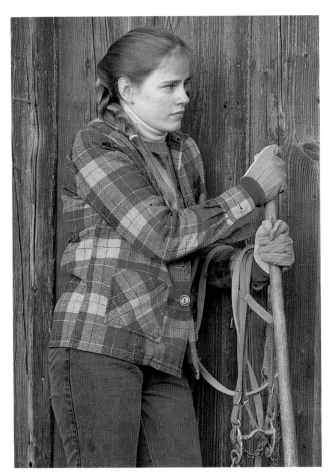

cord blue on film because they are illuminated by blue skylight, not sunlight. Consequently, whatever is photographed in shadows becomes contaminated with blue light, which creates a feeling of emotional distance in a photograph. ◆ I moved Amy to a new location where she was bathed in early morning sunlight. The colors created in this composition are more inviting to the eye, and the warm light invites the viewer to participate emotionally with the subject.

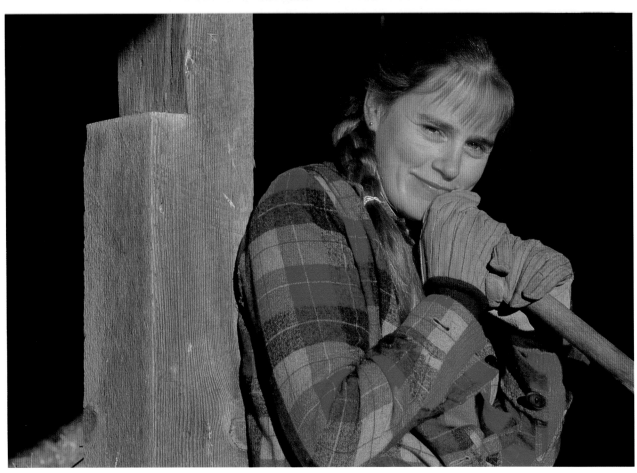

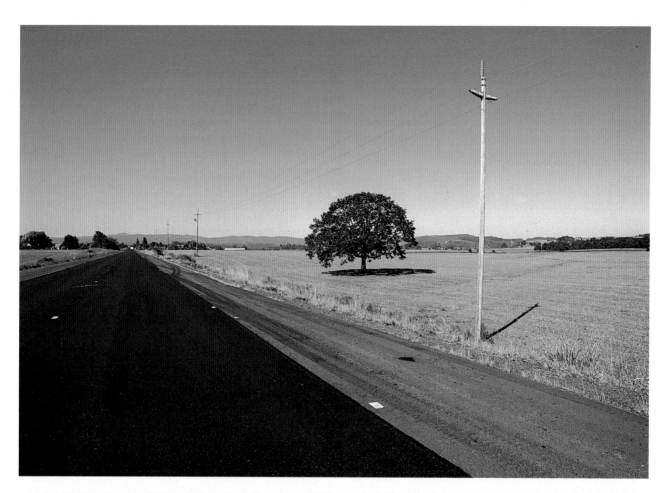

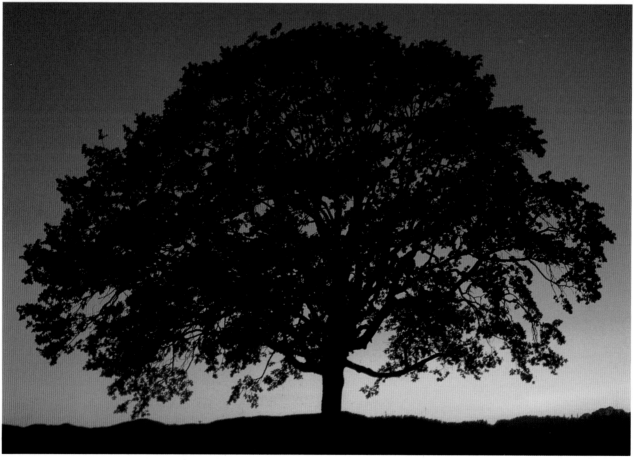

I love to shoot oak trees, perhaps because they symbolize great strength and determination or maybe because there are so many of them in the fields and hills near my home. The solitary oak you see in these pictures grows beside a highway near Banks, Oregon. I have returned to this oak countless times, to shoot it under different lighting and weather conditions at all times of the day.

◆ One night following sunset I put my 50mm lens and camera on a tripod and exposed the oak for 8 seconds. This silhouetted the oak against a beautiful continuum of colors. ◆ Later that summer after the wheat harvest, I returned to the oak early one morning. I was able to back up against its trunk and with my 20mm lens shoot its long shadow cascading across the stubble in front of me. ◆ At winter's first snowfall, I found my oak standing proud despite torturous, subfreezing temperatures. With my 105mm lens and camera firmly mounted on a tripod, I chose a shutter speed of 1/60 sec. to record the action of the falling snow as a slight blur. I then adjusted my aperture until a one-stop overexposure was indicated.

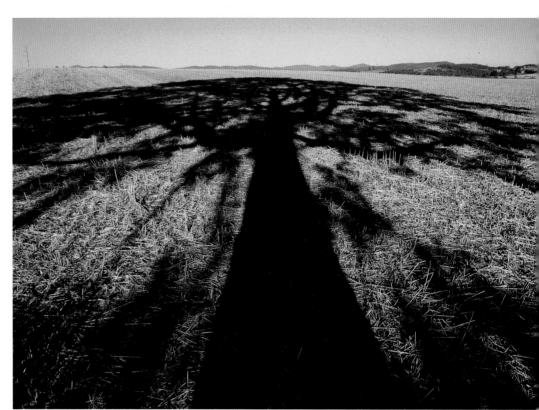

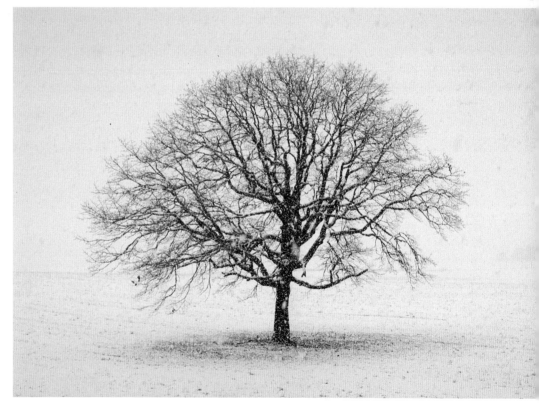

Shooting from Dawn to Dusk

The color of daylight varies according to the time of day and the weather. The midday sun produces a white light that begins a few hours after sunrise and lasts until a few hours before sunset. The overhead direction and colorless quality of midday light make this time of day the least likely to produce dramatic photographs, which is why so many professional photographers prefer to shoot early and late in the day. (Early morning light is the purest because much of the previous work day's pollution has since settled to the ground.) Just before dawn and for about an hour after sunset, cool, blue skylight casts an air of mystery across the landscape. At sunrise this light is replaced by a much warmer part of the spectrum, and for the next hour a golden light bathes frontlit and sidelit subjects in gold, orange, and red colors that arouse a warm response in the viewer. The same process occurs in reverse an hour before sunset, after which daylight quickly becomes blue skylight and again envelops the landscape in cool hues. For many photographers, this marks the end of the day, which is unfortunate because twilight can create a wonderful, enigmatic feeling in a photograph.

When the sun is low in the sky, your subject will either be frontlit, backlit, or sidelit, depending on your camera position. It has a profound effect on the moods you can create with available light. Frontlighting occurs when the sun is at your back. If you face a subject in the west at dawn or in the east at sunset, your camera will record vivid colors of orange and gold. A frontlit city skyline reflecting the sunrise is a particularly dramatic subject. The mood of the picture will be intensified if the city is showcased against the dark background of a passing storm. Frontlit landscapes do pose a major problem for wide-angle lenses because a low-angled sun at your back will cast a long shadow of you across the landscape. Due to the wide, sweeping vision of the wide-angle lens, your composition will suffer from your shadow's intrusion. Assuming you don't want your shadow recorded, you must either wait until the sun moves higher in the sky to be rid of it or switch to a normal or telephoto lens.

Backlighting occurs when you face the sun. Most backlit compositions render their subjects as silhouettes with bold shapes and stark outlines. Although silhouettes appear to be simple compositions, they are in fact among the most difficult to do correctly. The potential for objects to merge, which was discussed earlier in "Composing Strong Photographs," can only be avoided by careful attention and careful metering. To make silhouettes during sunsets and sunrises, you'll need to *increase* your exposure one stop beyond the indicated reading to ensure correct exposure. As a technique for silhouetting subjects, backlighting isn't limited to sunrises or sunsets; it can also be used at midday. For example, you might see rows of blackbirds perched along powerlines in the sky. You could move under the lines and frame the birds against the midday sun. The silhouettes resulting from the birds' underexposure are likely to create an impression similar to a moonlit scene.

Because leaves and feathers are transparent, they are also good subjects for strong backlight. Imagine walking along the beach and picking up a feather. Then with your macro lens and camera on a tripod, hold the feather several inches from the lens. Shift your point of view until the feather is bathed in the sun's strong backlight. Its illuminating effect on the intricate details of the feather's texture and shape will be breathtaking.

Of the three lighting conditions—frontlight, backlight, and sidelight—sidelight is by far the most dramatic for recording detail and color in your subjects. Sidelighting occurs when you shoot north or south at right angles to a low-angled sun in early morning or late afternoon. This generates an exciting tension between the deep tones and the bright highlights in the resulting photographs. Sidelighting a subject produces long shadows that bring a wonderful sense of depth to a scene, and this kind of light is the best for emphasizing a subject's texture.

On assignment for a hydropower company, I was sent to photograph McNary Dam on the border between Oregon and Washington. Several hours after my arrival, I felt I'd found an exciting composition with my 24mm lens by lying on a concrete abutment at the edge of a small puddle. However, the light was anything but flattering. A storm seemed to be entrenched directly overhead and threatened to prevent any possibility of shooting the dam in the golden light of late afternoon. ◆ How important are persistence and a dose of luck? Four hours later the clouds parted in the western sky. The last rays of the sun bathed the dam in golden light, making it look like a gold trophy instead of a gray monolith.

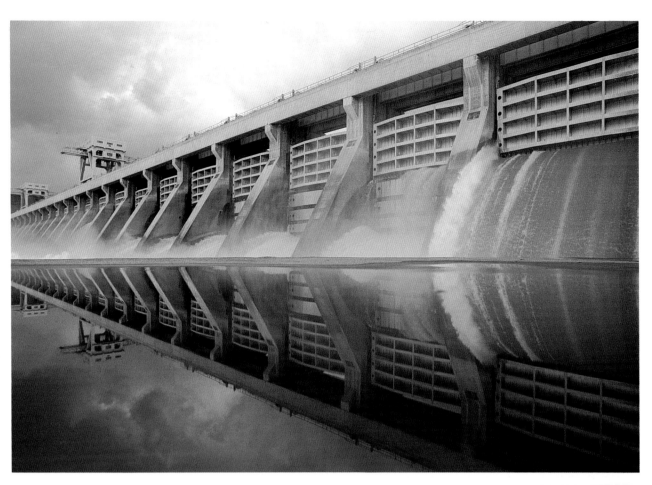

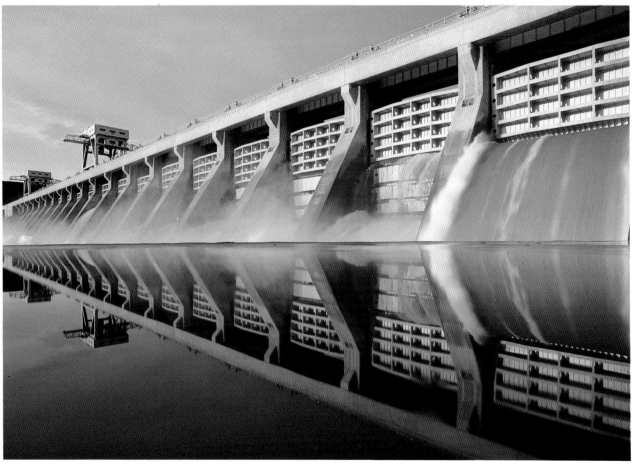

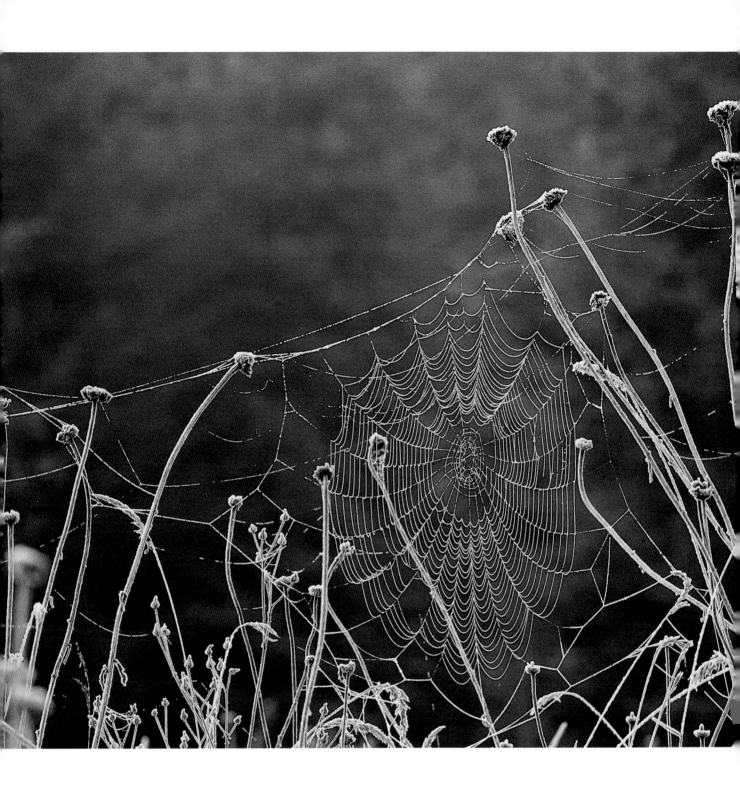

LEARNING
TO SEE
CREATIVELY

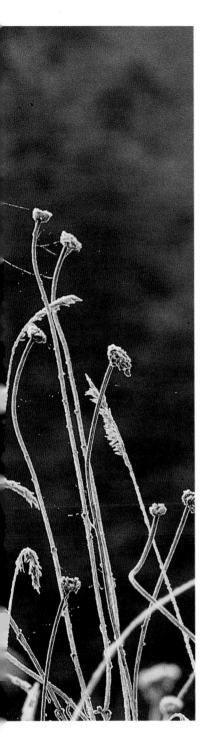

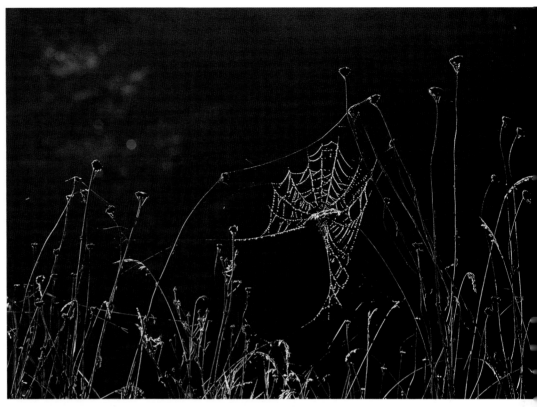

Arriving at one of my favorite meadows, I spotted numerous spider webs covered by a thick frost. Because the meadow was in a small valley, the early morning sun had yet to reach it, but it was filled with blue skylight from the clear sky overhead. I knew the blue light would enhance the mood of the frost-covered webs, since both frost and the color blue elicit the sensation of cold in viewers. ◆ Moving quickly with my 200mm lens and a 36mm extension tube, I chose this frozen web to convey the feeling of the cold morning. After I shot only nine exposures, the sun appeared, and its heat quickly turned the frost to dew. Had I arrived at this point, I would have missed the marvelous, frozen composition I found simply by getting up early.

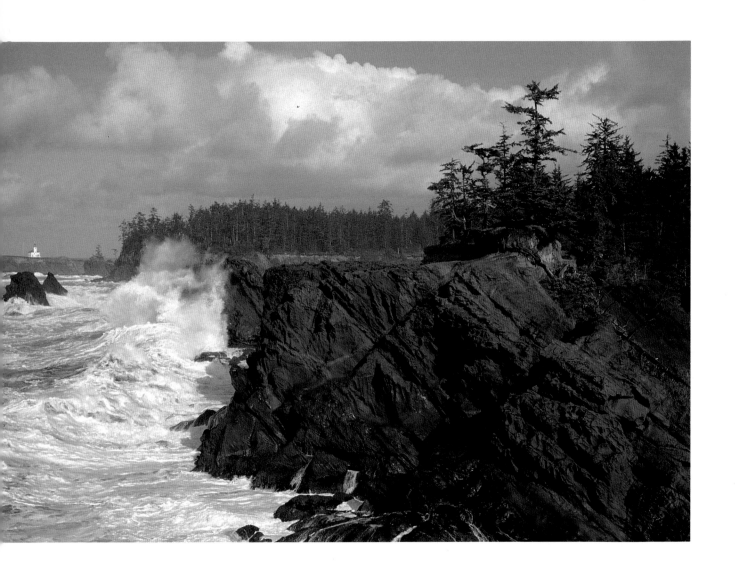

One of the world's most beautiful beaches stretches along Oregon's central coastline. Combining the beauty of Shore Acres State Park with the visual impact of Cape Arago's lighthouse created this remarkable composition. By day its colors, crashing surf, and textures are readily identified, but following sunset, the composition becomes very mysterious, even peaceful. Setting my 50mm lens at f/22 enabled me to make a 60-second exposure. Such a long exposure time will transform any crashing surf into an ethereal bed of calm. ◆ Making a long exposure at this time of day is perhaps easier than you think. First you set your lens wide open and adjust your shutter speed until your exposure meter says you've reached a correct exposure. If you're using ISO 100 film, your shutter speed will probably be around ½ or 1 second. Now close your lens down at least four stops. Assuming you are using a lens with a maximum aperture of f/2.8, you would stop down four stops to f/11. Since you've decreased the light transmission by four stops, you now need to increase your exposure time by four stops to maintain correct exposure; so you would need a shutter speed of 16 seconds, assuming your starting exposure was for 1 second. ◆ With your camera firmly mounted on a tripod, set the shutter-speed dial to 'B,' and use your locking cable release to hold the shutter open for 16 seconds. If you want to shoot for 32 seconds, set your aperture to f/16. If you want to shoot for 60 seconds, set your aperture to f/22. The longer you expose crashing surf, the calmer it will appear to be.

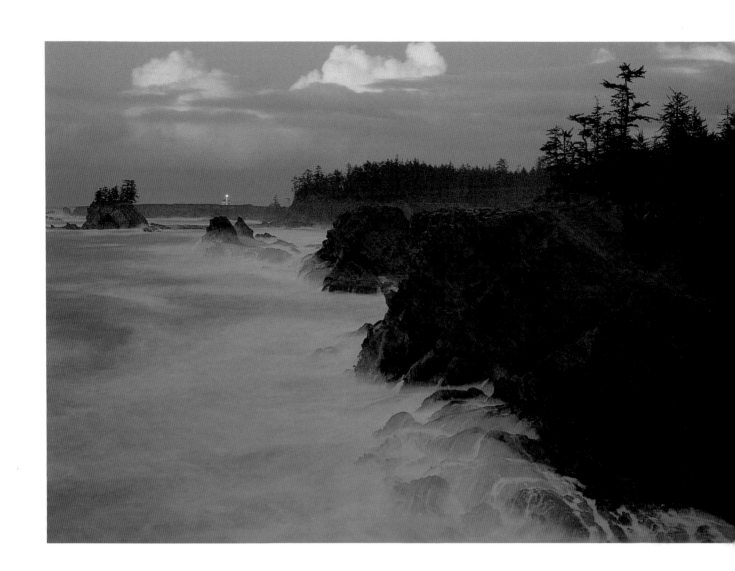

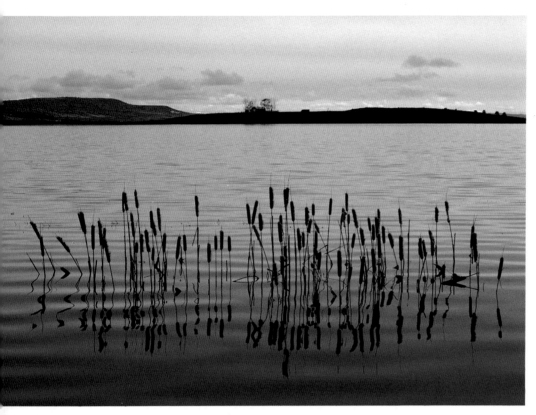

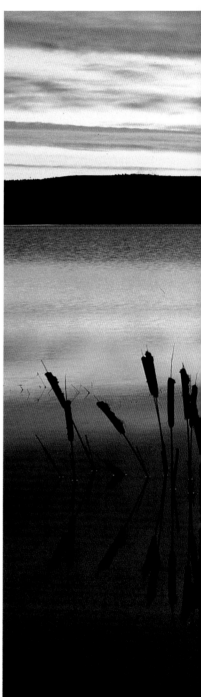

After a brief discussion with a nearby farmer, I was assured that these cattails, the lake, and a distant homestead would be backlit by the early morning sunrise—assuming, of course, that the next day's weather proved more fruitful than the storm overhead. ◆ That night in my motel room I set my alarm to go off forty-five minutes before sunrise, giving me enough time to return to this location for the hoped-for photograph. Brief as the sunrise was, it remains one of my all-time favorites. Within several minutes the storm closed off the dawn light, and soon it began to rain again. Returning to my car, I looked back at the landscape and tipped my hat in thanks for the brief respite.

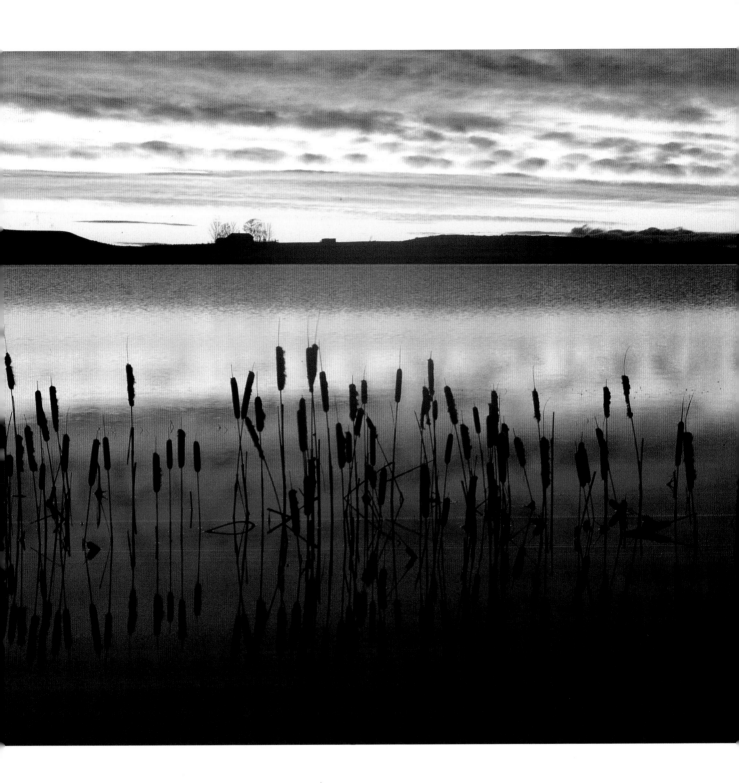

The Advantage of Overcast

Despite the warm, inviting appeal of gold light, don't become so seduced by it that you find yourself shooting only on clear days in the early morning or late afternoon. Many opportunities to create other moods with your subjects rely heavily on lighting conditions that are far from perfect. Clear days are not the only times to compose effective and powerful photographs. Diffused light caused by rain, mist, fog, or snow may conjure the best mood for presenting your subject. Some subjects simply don't come to life without the light created by weather conditions that nonphotographers find depressing.

The soft light of a cloudy day is excellent for capturing special moods in nature and in portraits. Beneath an overcast sky the entire spectrum of colors is much richer. If you need to prove this to yourself, go out to your garden and shoot some flowers on a sunny day and on a cloudy day. Your film will prove that color is more vivid when sunlight is diffused by clouds. Forests are especially exciting on cloudy days because the sharp contrast between well-lit areas and deep shadows is eliminated, which simplifies ex-

posures and makes colors softer and richer. An overcast day also extends the tonal range. Acting like a giant umbrella, the soft light of an overcast day produces the most flattering portraits, whether posed or candid. Faces appear softer and kinder whenever they are photographed out of the sun's direct light.

Rainy, foggy, misty, and snowy days are also good times to experiment with light. An old farmstead photographed in snow or against a gathering storm conveys much more drama than when photographed frontlit on a sunny day. In snow scenes variations of color and tone merge into subtle gradations of black, gray, and white, creating an almost ethereal quality. And in rain, mist, or fog subjects appear to lose their hard edges, which softens their shapes and lend an air of mystery to compositions. If you're using your camera on automatic in such situations, then set your autoexposure dial to +1 or 2×. For manual exposures, adjust your aperture or shutter speeds until a one-stop overexposure is indicated. This will eliminate gray snow or dark fog caused by the camera meter's tendency toward underexposure.

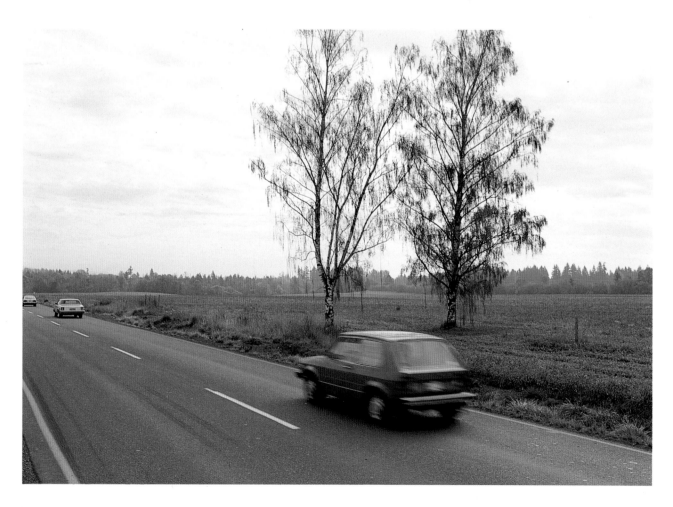

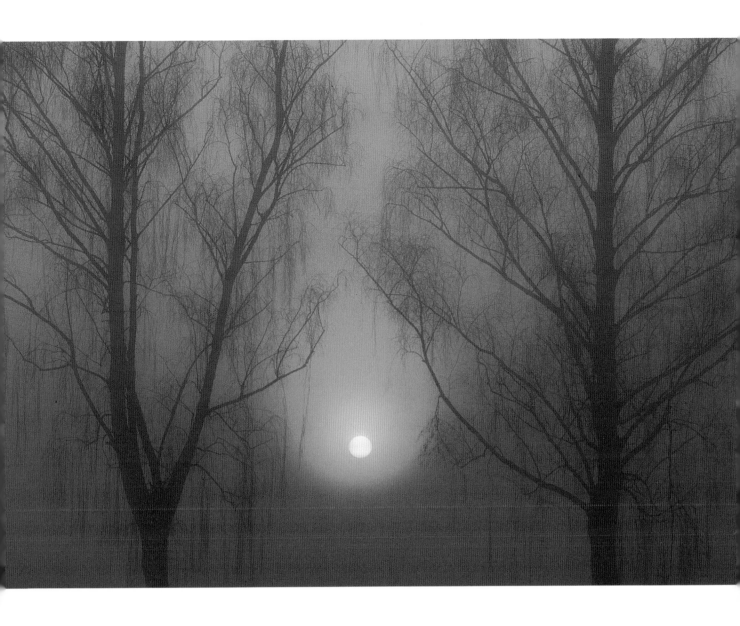

I had driven past these two birch trees countless times and had never paid any attention to them until one morning when I came upon them in the fog. Once again, I was rewarded for carrying my equipment with me at all times. Without hesitation I parked on the road's shoulder and hastily mounted my 105mm lens and camera on a tripod. Firing quickly, I was able to make four exposures of the morning sun rising through a thin veil of fog.

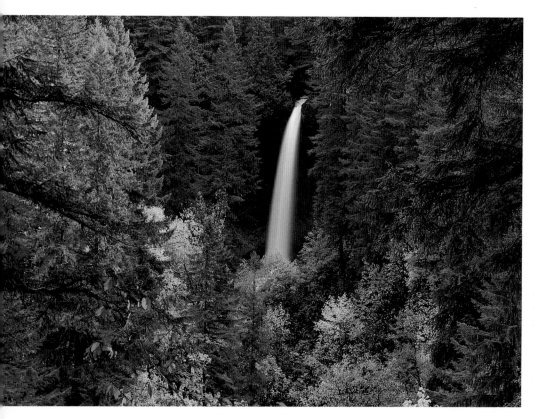

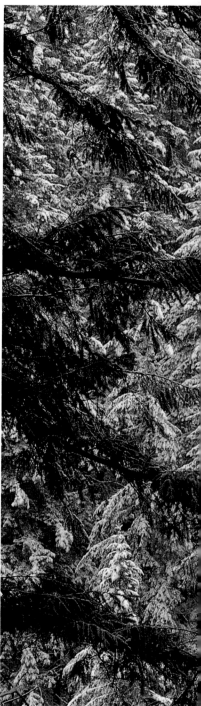

I have been to Silver Falls State Park, east of Salem, Oregon, many times during the past five years but only once during a snowfall. Fresh snowfall always casts a wonderful silence over any landscape and transforms worn-out compositions into fresh, exciting visions. Like many other photographers, I've stood at this bend in the road and shot the North Falls in spring, summer, and autumn. However, until this snowfall I was never pleased with my results. ◆ To make this picture I mounted my camera and 105mm lens securely on a tripod, set my aperture to *f*/22, and prefocused the scene via the depth-of-field scale. Then I adjusted my shutter speed until a one-stop overexposure was indicated.

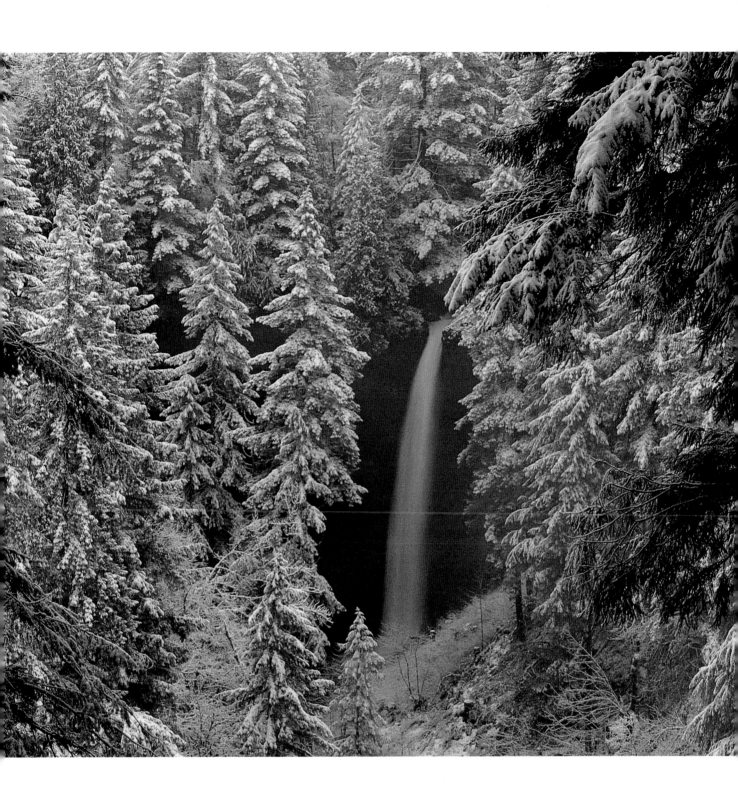

INDEX

142 | LEARNING
     TO SEE
     CREATIVELY

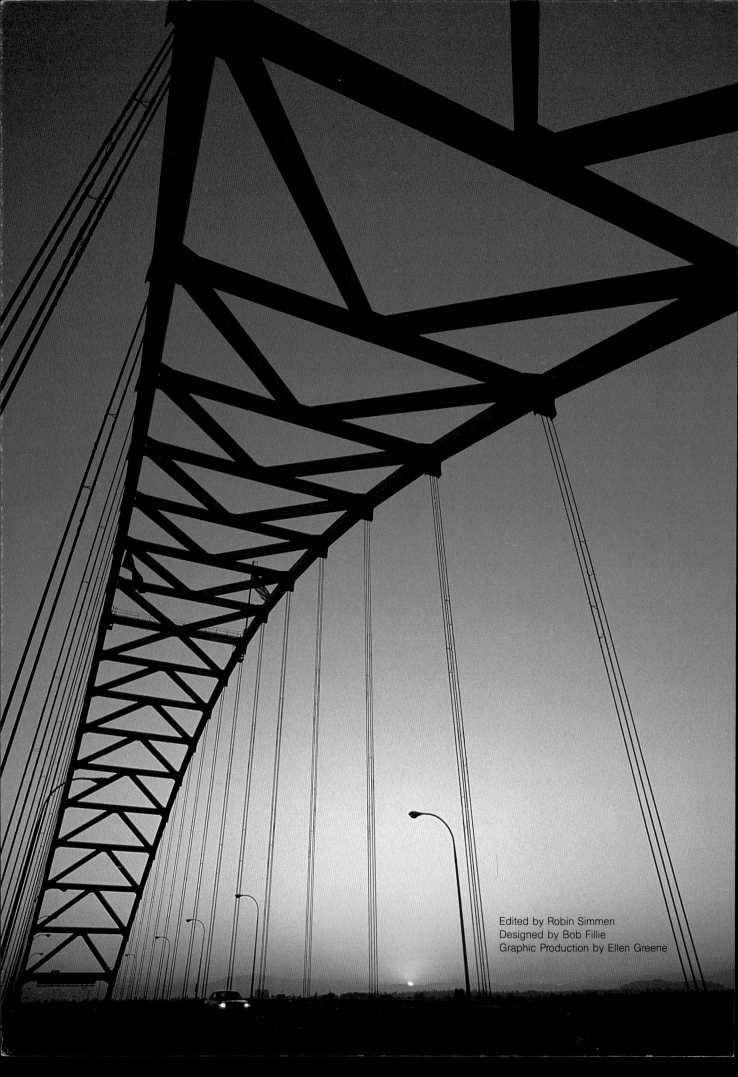

Edited by Robin Simmen
Designed by Bob Fillie
Graphic Production by Ellen Greene